THE DUDES' GUIDE TO PREGNANCY

Dealing with Your Expecting Wife, Coming Baby, and the End of Life as You Knew It

Bill Lloyd *and* Scott Finch

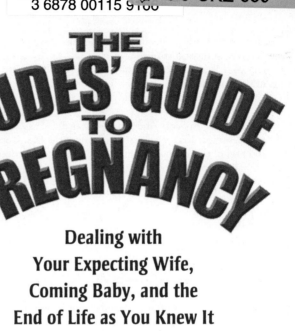

WELLNESS CENTRAL

NEW YORK   BOSTON

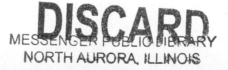

The advice herein is not intended to replace the services of trained health professionals, or be a substitute for medical advice. You are advised to consult with your health care professional with regard to matters relating to your health, and in particular regarding matters that may require diagnosis or medical attention.

Wellness Central
Hachette Book Group USA
237 Park Avenue
New York, NY 10017

Visit our Web site at www.HachetteBookGroupUSA.com.

Wellness Central is an imprint of Grand Central Publishing.
The Wellness Central name and logo are trademarks of Hachette Book Group USA, Inc.

Printed in the United States of America

First Edition: May 2008
10 9 8 7 6 5 4 3 2 1

Library of Congress Cataloging-in-Publication Data

Finch, Scott.
    The dudes' guide to pregnancy : dealing with your expecting wife, coming baby, and the end of life as you knew it / Scott Finch & Bill Lloyd.—1st ed.
        p. cm.
    Includes index.
    ISBN-13: 978-0-446-17819-8
    ISBN-10: 0-446-17819-5
    1. Pregnancy—Popular works.   2. Husbands.   I. Lloyd, Bill, 1976–
II. Title.
    RG556.F56 2008
    618.2—dc22
                                                                2007027360

For years, our wives, Jessie and Amy, told us that we were funny and attractive. We never believed them. However, the publication of this book proves that they were at least half right. This book is dedicated to them.

Acknowledgments

We would sincerely like to thank David Kuhn and Billy Kingsland at Kuhn Projects for their expert advice, motivation, and belief in The Dudes. We literally could not have done this without you.

We would also like to thank Diana Baroni for her expert editing and infinite patience (even while pregnant). And Alison Bonaguro for her constant encouragement/nagging to actually finish this project.

We would especially like to thank all of our friends who unwittingly provided material and didn't know we were writing a book. You guys are the best.

Contents

Foreword

Welcome to the first sentence of the most important book you'll ever read in your whole entire life. We are The Dudes. Our names are Bill Lloyd and Scott Finch, but we are so much more than that. We are a combination of your grandfather, your father, your friends (not the dumb ones), and anyone else who dispenses helpful advice for the purpose of making you less stupid. We, like you, enjoy fried foods, electronic gadgets, professional sports, and "your mom" jokes. We are the oversight committee for any self-respecting man and are dedicated to the relentless pursuit of totally kicking ass. Any dude can join us and become one of The Dudes, but none of those "I have a penis but was born with the soul of a woman" males are welcome...yeesh. We don't have time to hear about your sensitivity issues, because the pregame is about to begin. We offer advice, make decrees, and belittle you when you deserve it (which is more often than you think, dumbass).

The Dudes recognize that manhood is a big tent, and men of any race, religion, social status, or economic standing are welcome (and if you have money to spring for the pizza, that'll help). After all, it is our differences that make

us great, unless of course those differences are vegetarianism or a love of professional soccer.

Importantly, The Dudes recognize that propagation of
the species is essential to our own existence. We understand that there is a hard way and an easy way to deal with
pregnancy—a right way and a wrong way. We understand
that the experience can be a difficult and arduous one for
men. The Dudes' first and foremost recommendation is a
universal one:

"Suck it up and bury your feelings deep, deep down
inside."

While the suggestions in this book are all very useful, be
advised they are all ancillary to the above suggestion.

On behalf of self-respecting men everywhere, The Dudes
wish you Godspeed.

Introduction

It's God's gift to humanity. It's your legacy. It's Nature's perfect parasite.

Bill remembers the day his wife took her pregnancy test. It was beautiful, special, historic…and *hilarious*! That's mostly because, if you look at the instructions that come with the pregnancy test, you'll see an artist's rendering of a lady peeing on a stick. Seriously, a drawing of a woman peeing? It doesn't get any funnier than that and should keep you laughing for the next three to four minutes as you wait for two pink lines, a plus sign, or the rabbit injected with your wife's urine to gasp for its last breath of sweet, life-giving oxygen.[1]

Anyway, the test was positive. Bill and his wife embraced as his laughter quickly turned to tears, which he assured his wife were tears of joy (which she *totally* bought).

It was a great moment for both of them. She looked forward to nine months of attention and being cute, and Bill made a pact with himself not to take for granted the last 280 days (403,200 minutes) of life as he knew it.

He was fortunate enough to have a good friend, Scott, who had become a father months before him. Scott's wife,

---

1. Applies to Arkansas residents only.

a teacher turned stay-at-home mom, gave Bill's wife, a teacher and soon-to-be stay-at-home mom, the lowdown on the wonderful journey she was about to embark on. Similarly, Scott gave Bill biweekly briefings on what emotions, needs, dodging of flying objects (including toast[2]), and general awfulness to expect. The following ten chapters are those briefings and are our $12 gift to you... *The Dudes' Guide to Pregnancy*. If you have half as much fun reading this book as we did writing it, we will have enjoyed this book twice as much as you.

Checklist

As you begin your forty-week adventure, realize that a lot of what will happen can easily be dealt with on a learn-as-you-go basis. However, there are several situations that The Dudes' experience and expertise will help you avoid. To maximize the book's usefulness, we have compiled a list of essential items you will need for the next nine months. We suggest you procure the following items as quickly as possible:

- *alcohol:* In any drinkable form. It truly takes the edge off. Alternate suggestions include Prozac, Zoloft, Paxil, Wellbutrin, Lexapro, lithium, or any other medication Tom won't let Katie take.
- *one medium-sized monkey:* A well-trained ape can take care of several tasks you would not want to do yourself. Midgets are a suitable substitute but are harder to housebreak.

---

2. As explained in detail in chapter 2.

- *ten to twelve large rubber bands*
- *pirate costume:* Trust us, you'll need it (for the hard times).
- *2 tablespoons fresh basil*

Note: One important item missing from the list above is dignity. That is not a mistake. You will not need any and will consequently be hard-pressed to find even a shred for months, nay years, to come.

People Who Shouldn't Read This Book

This book is strictly intended for *male reading only.* The subject matter is privileged, private, and confidential and is explicitly not intended for a female audience. Please understand that sharing the information herein with women would make Pandora's box look like a Rubik's Cube. You don't want to be responsible for opening that can of worms, do you?

As a precaution, this book is equipped with the latest in secure publishing technology. The cover and pages are coated with a harmful chemical agent that is activated by the pH exclusive to a woman's skin. In laboratory tests, the resulting chemical reaction has caused severe skin deformities, making test subjects appear to resemble Joan Rivers...ew. Consider yourself warned.

Note to Those Who Knocked Up Girlfriends

This book is written in the context of heterosexuals conceiving children in holy wedlock. However, we feel the topics are mostly universal to pregnant women and their sperm-donating counterparts. Yes, we feel it can be a good read even if you are reading from the comfort of your parents' basement, with your baby's mamma next to you on the futon.

It's important you know that we do not judge those who have children out of wedlock. We'll leave it to the Almighty to send you to hell to burn for eternity.

Enjoy.

B.C.
Before Conception

This is going to be easy.

If you paid attention when your high school gym teacher was awkwardly explaining the process of conception in health class, then you're familiar with the way in which a single sperm fertilizes an egg. Or perhaps Coach used a garbled filmstrip or video to explain it to you, since he was likely busy planning an airtight strategy for the homecoming game or covering up the sexual relationship he was having with one of your classmates. Either way, if you're not sure how conception works, a different book or the opening sequence of *Look Who's Talking* could explain it better than we can. Our purpose is not to give you a boner (that's what the Internet is for). Rather, as the title of our book suggests, we, The Dudes, are here to guide you down the path of twenty-first-century pregnancy. We're here to give you The Dudes' point of view, something sorely lacking in all the other pregnancy primers out there, almost all of which are aimed at your wife.

The fact that you're reading this book indicates that you're in the process of planning to impregnate some female. Or that your wife recently told you that you knocked her up, and you've come crawling to us for answers. Either way, like a good friend, we're reluctantly here for you. Unlike a good friend, though, we plan to be honest and forthright. Whereas your toadying friends might tell you that your five-alarm chili tastes great or that your band is "fun to listen to," we will tell you that your band is lame and your chili tastes like a dead hooker's butt. That's right, no sugar coating here.

We understand that many men may not want to know the truth. They would like to be surprised by the wondrous changes wrought by pregnancy on their wives' bodies; they want to discover for themselves the emerging fountains of life before them. We, The Dudes, completely understand, and would even like to help those men by offering a list of alternate resources for them and their "partners."

Pregnant and Loving It, by Alice Baker-Ornelas
Your Vagina Loves You, by Joan Dietz-Debello
Vaginas, Vaginas, Vaginas, by Gertrude "Dr. Gerty"
    Bending-Mansfield, PhD
You and Your Wuss Husband, by Carol Salzman-
    Peterson

If you truly want to sympathize with the nausea, exhaustion, and misery your wife will experience during her pregnancy, simply read a few pages of one of these pregnancy books for chicks (a few chapters will induce vomiting). Here is some actual text from actual women's pregnancy literature:

Consider what you're getting and not what you're los-ing. Your new roundness provides more surface area for your lover to see and touch. Any time you feel yourself falling back into your old mindset, call a friend who's been there and ask her to talk you out of it. Stand in front of a mirror and embrace the new version of your-self. Take pride in your "new" body—give it the respect it deserves. (from www.askdrsears.com)

Feel free to take a moment to choke back the bile rising in your throat. Consider what you're getting?!? You're *getting* pounds, about forty-five of them. Take pride in yourself? We heard a 400-pound lady saying the same thing on *Oprah* the other day. We actually did a tally and found eighty-seven things wrong with the above passage.

Women's pregnancy books are all about women appreciating their new selves, celebrating their sebaceous glands, savoring their stretch marks, exalting in their expanding asses. The Dudes frown strongly upon such I'm-okay, you're-okay psychobabble. Don't get us wrong, however—as part of our credo of strict honesty, we'd be lying if we told you that telling the truth is always a good idea. A well-placed lie—or, from the Latin for false truth, *reproba verum*—is one of the art forms of pregnancy and can play a vital role in your survival. "No, baby, those jeans don't look like they would scream if they had the capacity to communicate pain," is one of many *reproba vera* that will help liberate you from the awkwardness of truthfulness.

We have done the research and can tell you with confidence that every sentence of every women's pregnancy book is complete bunk. Whatever the advice, be it practical ("Use a rubber band when you can't button those jeans anymore"), emotional ("Just think of your teary outbursts as practice for happy tears when your baby is finally born"), spiritual ("God knows what She's doing"), or otherwise ("Real women have stretch marks"), rest assured, it's crappity crap. We even found a broad's book that claims you can influence the gender of your baby through the sexual position you use during coitus. Here are some tried-and-untrue, no-nonsenseless methods for porking your way to preferred chromosomes:

If you want a boy:

- make love standing up.
- try the rear-entry position.
- focus on his pleasure—if the male partner climaxes first, you're guaranteed a boy.
- mark your calendar—more boys are conceived on odd days of the month.

If you want a girl:

- give the missionary position a go.
- make love with the woman on top.
- focus on her pleasure—if the woman orgasms before her partner, you can decorate your nursery in pink.
- get together on the even days of the month.

The Dudes can assure you the above methods boast a remarkable 50 percent success rate and that this nonsense hocus-pocus is about as useful as Wicca, voodoo, and kabbalah.

Into the Great Wide Open

Back in the fourth grade, a new kid came to school. He was a pompous know-it-all and bully who used to hold kids down and spit into their mouths at recess. We liked him right away. He taught us things we'd never seen or heard of before, some boring, some brilliant. Since then, we've managed to keep this good friend, Science, at arm's length, using him only when absolutely necessary. He's helpful when we need him but can be a pain in the ass when he has to get in an unwelcome word (just ask the "intelligent design" folks about that). One great thing is nowadays, we can get him drunk and manipulate him into saying just about anything we want, to help us win an argument. Unfortunately, we have to follow a precise procedure to get him to do our bidding. This process is known as the scientific method. It usually starts with beer and segues into shots and casual drug use, as necessary.

Anyway, the smartest guy we know, Science, tells us that a full-term pregnancy lasts about nine months, or forty weeks. However, if the practice of lobotomies and that whole "round-earth" hoax have taught us anything, it's that he may have gotten into his secret cache of 'shrooms again. From The Dudes' perspective, pregnancy begins the moment your wife decides she wants to have a baby, which can tack on anywhere from one week to a full year of misery to the forty weeks you've been told about. In fact, most OB/GYNs will tell you it can take up to a year to get pregnant, so your pregnancy "journey" can easily last nearly two years. And like the great historical journeys of Odysseus, Lewis and Clark, and the Griswold family, the pregnancy journey is often wrought with adventure, peril, surprises, the Cyclops, fur trading, and naked Christie Brinkley in a pool.

The process begins innocently enough. "Let's have a baby," your wife might say to you with an anxious smile. Then she'll throw away the birth control pills, and you do something that, up until this point, you've never done in your entire life: you have sex with a woman for the purpose of making her pregnant. Let's think about this for a second: for the past one to thirty-five years, you've been fornicating knowing that a certain possibility lurks in the background, the possibility that she could get knocked up, the unfortunate side effect of gettin' some. Suddenly, the entire concept of sex as you have known it is turned on its ear. From your first peek at a poorly hidden *Playboy* or *Hustler,* sex has existed to give you a reason to exist. It has vexed you, embraced you, and embarrassed you with little regard for your well-being. Sex was something that most of your life's important moments were defined by.

So now that you are for the first time in your life *trying* to get a woman pregnant, sex has become a means by which the male of the species fertilizes a woman's egg for purposes of procreation. All at once the notion of sex being forbidden is gone. The idea that the neighbors might look out and see you doing it on the back lawn is a thing of the past. The image of getting it on in a 90-degree Porta John at the NASCAR race (hello, Southern readers!) is a sweaty, smelly memory. The inevitable has arrived, and although you won't be having sex like a porn star anymore, you'll be having sex as often as a porn star for weeks or months to come.

Like a bathroom remodel that you thought was going to be a quick two- or three-day project, all of a sudden it's six months later, and you still haven't put up the baseboard. One night in the bedroom, after ejaculating air, you realize, "Ohhhh, it takes a while." Listen closely to yourself— that's the sound of you realizing you've been wrong about everything. Like remember when you thought your wife was mad at you because you ate that whole box of chocolates without sharing, but it turns out she was mad because you actually bought the chocolates for her? Or that time you were supposed to go buy a new refrigerator but came home with an HD DVR instead because it would "practically pay for itself"? Yep, you have a long and prosperous history of being wrong. It's nice that you've finally discovered this

Infancy: You suckled at your mother's breast. Can't figure out why you're a boob man, huh, Oedipus?

Grade School: The extent to which a girl was infected with "cooties" determined your relationship with her.

Middle School: You chose not to give that important speech to the class because of your spontaneous adolescent erection.

Homecoming: You found a date who had the best odds of letting you stick your hands down her pants.

College: You went to the school with the most hot chicks and often skipped working on important papers to go to parties to meet girls.

Religion: "God, please don't let her be pregnant."

Relationships: When you decided to get married, the phrase "Is this the one woman I want to have sex with for the rest of my life?" was an important part in your decision-making process.

Career: Whenever the hot temp or intern is in the building, your productivity halves.

yourself, as your wife will be reminding you of this for at least the next nine months.

As your sex life becomes less and less maniacal and more and more mechanical, the transformation continues. In your younger days, after sex, you prayed that your girlfriend/chick you met at the bar wasn't pregnant. You remember the prayer that started "Dear God, I don't know if you're out there, but if you are…" and ended "…and if you can do this one thing for me, I'll never have sex again." It was a holy prayer of desperation, aka God's most ignored prayer.

As the former sex-craving you starts to die inside, you might actually start to look forward to your wife's absence of a period. You and your tired unit may even rejoice when the first day of her cycle comes and goes with no sign of…ugh, you know. Then your wife becomes pregnant. You may jump up and down for joy, but you should do so with caution, because The Dudes have some things to warn you about.

Missed Conceptions

Miscarriage, or "divine abortion," is an almost inevitable part of early pregnancy. As a male, you can accept that fact and place it on your list of things to be wary of—you know, the list that also contains the following things to be wary of:

- stock tips
- poison ivy/oak
- French cuisine
- snakes with red, black, and yellow stripes (after all, red next to yellow *can* kill a fellow)
- your wife saying, "Honey, what's this?" or "We need to talk."

■ starting a conversation with the computer guy at work
■ girls with Adam's apples

The female perspective on miscarriages is radically different, however. To your wife, a bundle of cells that has formed in her uterus during the first couple weeks is her unborn child with whom she is instantly in love. The new hormones that quickly begin to circulate throughout her body reinforce this bond, and the longer you've been trying to get pregnant, the stronger this bond is. As much as a miscarriage is almost inevitable, so is the prospect of it being a wholly heartfelt and genuinely upsetting experience for your wife. What makes it so strange is your almost certain disconnect from the entire situation. Sure you're upset, but only because your wife is upset. After all, these things happen. The Dudes suggest supporting her through her tears and reminding her that someday soon you'll have a beautiful, kick-ass baby. Plus, you'll have just enough of a break from sex for the chafing to heal.

Given that the miscarriage was a pretty significant event in her life, your wife will likely tell her mom, sister, and close friends about it. They will inevitably offer one of the following five nuggets of wisdom:

1. "Maybe it wasn't meant to be."
2. "Things always work out for the best."
3. "When one door closes, another one opens."
4. "Time heals all wounds."

...and, our personal favorite,

5. "Everything happens for a reason."

Despite their fatuous clichés, your wife's friends will be able to offer her *way* better emotional support than whatever you can come up with. Yeah, this would be a good time to keep to yourself your theory about how the miscarriage may actually be a good thing because the embryo might have been messed up, so her body wisely rejected it, even though Science says your theory is pretty sound. You wife's mood will get better, and soon you'll start having that mechanical sex again. But the miscarriage will have one lasting side-effect: the secret fact that you've been trying to get pregnant is now out. Despite your wife's upsetting experience, your mother-in-law and/or sister-in-law are secretly celebrating, because now they know about the *trying*. Now you're on Pregnancy Watch.

Pregnancy Watch is the term The Dudes coined to describe the situation that arises when all of your wife's friends and family know she is trying to get knocked up. As bizarre as it might sound to those of you who haven't experienced this, your friends and family will actually follow your wife's monthly cycle. This means that they'll constantly be asking her (or you) if she got her period this month. The idea of a Dude's mother-in-law asking his wife about her period reminds us of a TV commercial for tampons and actually gives *us* a "not-so-fresh" feeling.

The Mother-in-Law

You know all those jokes and humorous anecdotes that you've always heard about mothers-in-law? You know, like "My mother-in-law got bit by a dog yesterday. She's fine, but the dog died." The Dudes would like to remind to you that despite the fact that they may not be funny to anyone under the age of sixty, they're all true. "But my mother-in-law is really cool," you say. Like so many aspects of your life, things are about to change.

The mother-in-law is a master of manipulation. She is well versed in the Jedi mind trick and can convince you with a simple wave of the hand that "these aren't the droids you're looking for" or anything else to help her do her bidding in Mos Eisley or elsewhere. She is so good with manipulation, you often don't realize you're being manipulated. If you are aware, it's only because she wants you to be. She worships at the altar of The Great Know-It-All and regularly observes the holy sacrament of dispensing unsolicited advice.

"But my mother-in-law doesn't even know my wife's pregnant," you say. That's nice that you think that. Do you ever hear sounds in the middle of the night, sounds you can't explain? Listen while The Dudes make the unexplainable explainable. These are the sounds of one of your mother-in-law's favorite nighttime activities: rummaging through your garbage, your financial records, and even the bed you're lying in. She's that good.

Other favorite nighttime activities you may be unaware of include:

- barking/howling at the moon
- hunting for nightcrawlers (for a midnight snack)
- stalking, killing, skinning, drinking the blood of woodland creatures
- shaving her back
- knitting

Similarly, *your* mother will likely become your wife's nemesis. This relationship can often be much more antagonistic than your feud with her mom. Our friend Todd remembers a particularly cruel episode when his wife suffered her first miscarriage. She was, of course, devastated. Todd's mom was there to offer horrifying unsolicited advice to his tearful wife, such as, "Well, maybe if you didn't try to do so much work, the baby would have survived," or, "Hopefully, the next one will make it." Emotional scars have rarely run as deep or as wide. The mother-in-law's—yours or hers—wealth of advice doesn't stop there, though. She'll have little nuggets of demotivational wisdom to offer throughout the pregnancy.

☠   The Mother-in-Law Says   ☠

**"A miscarriage means that
you just didn't want it bad enough."**

Mother Load

Bill's knocking-up experience was decidedly un-unique. Once, during his junior year of high school, Bill's girlfriend was three weeks late and, despite having utilized elaborate methods of contraception, Bill was convinced that she was pregnant. Which led him to believe that he produced some sort of übersperm that could impregnate women in circumstances that other men's sperm would not. When Bill's girlfriend's monthly cycle caught up with her, Bill remained convinced of his übersperm's potency (as he does to this day) and believes that some sort of divine intervention was involved in his salvation.

When Bill's wife decided that she wanted to get pregnant, history had proven to Bill that this would be easy. She threw away her birth control pills, and a month later she was pregnant. But a month after that, she had a miscarriage. Okay, try again. One month later, not pregnant. Hrmm, must be something wrong with her. One month later, not pregnant again. Again, probably something wrong on her end.

When we humans finally acquire the technology to enable robots to have sex, Bill knows exactly how they will feel: "robo-fucking" became a daily occurrence over the next several months as he continued to try to impregnate his wife. You know the (true) expression "Sex is like pizza: even when it's bad it's still good"? Well, robo-fucking is kind of like pizza without the toppings, sauce, cheese, or dough. And like a job in human resources, it requires minimal effort, yet is mechanical and joyless. Robo-fucking is the opposite of "Hyatt Humping" (when on vacation, you get to do awesome stuff with your wife that you don't get to do at home)—it changes sex as you know it. It reminds you of your evolutionary purpose: sex is something you do to perpetuate the species as opposed to something you do to dirty hot chicks.

With an average 20 million sperm per helping, Bill estimated that approximately 3.8 billion sperm failed to do the one task assigned them. In a deeply honest moment of self-realization, it appeared that perhaps he was to blame for his lazy sperm. Bill knew it was likely his fault, as his sperm had been put through years of relentless self-induced partnerless ejaculation, conditioning the little guys not to accomplish the one task assigned them. The sky was now falling, but the townsfolk of Scrotum Falls (pop. 20 million) could no longer be convinced of that fact by the serial-masturbating Chicken Little. He had broken their will and, like middle management, expected them to pick up the slack and make him look good to his superiors (wife).

Somewhere in the midst of all this was the memory of the high school girlfriend and Bill's young, virile übersperm. He also jealously thought about all the burnout chicks that got knocked up so easily by their stoner boyfriends. Oh, and about the girl who heard you couldn't get pregnant the first time you had sex (who was already pregnant). Being a fan of both irony and sex, though, he could look back and laugh.

After a couple more months of his sperm doing just enough work to not get fired, the project was complete, and Bill's wife was pregnant. Everything was about to change.

Ask The Dudes

Dear Dudes,

My wife and I have been trying to get pregnant for MONTHS! We've tried all the tricks like oysters, sea urchin, and putting her ~~ass~~ legs up in the air, but it doesn't seem to be working!! She's been riding my ass DAY AND NIGHT about this. ~~Fucking~~ Sex is even starting to become a little monotonous. Any thoughts?

Sincerely,
Sea Man

Dear Sea,

You are *eating* the oysters and sea urchin, right? Unfortunately, weird Asian foods won't help make that one-in-20-million connection. So just relax, man, and maybe try something a little less slimy, like maybe...Uh-oh. We think we just heard your wife ovulating! Go get 'em, tiger!

Sincerely,

The Dudes

📖 Myth vs. Fact 📖

Myth: Women can get pregnant relatively easily.

Fact: Women you don't want to get pregnant can get pregnant relatively easily.

Myth: If you want to have a girl, make sure your wife climaxes first.

Fact: Married woman are actually incapable of achieving climax.

Myth: A woman will increase her odds of conception by elevating her pelvis and legs after sex.

Fact: A woman will increase her odds of conception by elevating her pelvis and legs after a gang bang.

CHAPTER ONE

Weeks 1–4

After several months of what can only be described as relentless porking, it's time to get your pregnancy on! The first indication is a late menstrual cycle. This can also coincide with nausea, irritability, and swollen breasts—among other things. Your wife may experience similar symptoms.

Urine Trouble

ATTENTION: Pregnancy tests cost about $20. Yeah, they cost a lot less your freshman year of college when your girlfriend was a week late and you swore to God you'd never have sex (or drink) again if she wasn't pregnant, only to toast your negative test result with a cold one and a quickie in the dorm later that night. But we're digressing. The prospect of such an expense this time around could make you think, "Do we really need to know *right now*?" I mean, if there's a baby in there, it ain't going anywhere, right?

Good luck with that.

A missed period used to be the first indicator that you got your wife knocked up. She missed a period. You bought a test. But recent technological innovations now allow for results a couple days before her period would otherwise have arrived. What this means to you is that you'll get to spend five to ten times more money on pregnancy tests than you would have a few short years ago. Thanks a lot, Science.

Here's the scenario. It's been three and a half solid weeks of nighttime fertilization. Your wife, excited by the prospect of being pregnant, buys a test. It's negative. Hrmmm, maybe she took it just a little too early. She buys another test. Negative. Hrmmmm, maybe she took it a little too early again. Repeat daily until her unwanted period arrives. Repeat previous steps every three and a half weeks until pregnant. You see how quickly this can add up?

Pregnancy tests also offer some benefits you won't find in the test instructions. They will work as a sort of litmus test for your wife's mood for the coming weeks. The Dudes like to call this the Groundhog Day effect: a negative result will mean three to four more weeks of frustration and anger; a positive test result will mean a brief period of elation, followed by nine months of frustration and anger.

If you're not yet out $40 to $400 for multiple pregnancy-test kits, you can do what The Dudes did: purchase the cheapy, generic, store-brand pregnancy test. It's just as easy for your wife to urinate on a Wal-vulation test or a Kroger Konception Kit as it is for her to urinate on an E.P.T.'s or your Clear Blue Easy's. That way you can use the money you saved to make a frivolous purchase, like a sweet new spoiler for the Subaru or a new toy for your soon-to-be-forgotten dog.

✓   **Pregnancy Test Quick Tip**   ✓

If the pregnancy test is negative, remember *she* is
supposed to supply the urine for the test—not you.
Now go try again.

Teamwork Makes a Team Work

Listen closely, because we're only going to say this once. You
don't ever, ever say, "My wife is pregnant," or "My wife
might be pregnant." If you had a clue what you were talking about, you would realize that although your wife may
indeed be pregnant, there's much more to it than that. Say
it with us, The Dudes, now: "*We're* pregnant." That's right.
Your wife's pregnant. You're pregnant. *We're* pregnant.

Awwwww, you think. She wants to include you in her
miraculous adventure, happily skipping down the nine-
month trail of life-giving happiness to arrive at the cute little cabbage patch to pick out your cherubic bundle of joy.
This is mostly true, but you have to change a few words.
Replace *miraculous adventure* with *unforgiving nightmare*, *happily skipping* with *awkwardly trundling*, *trail of
life-giving happiness* with *path to hell*, *cute little cabbage
patch* with *blood- and feces-spattered delivery room*, and
finally *pick out* with *painfully squeeze through your wife's
crotch*.

The expression *we're pregnant* is a not-so-subtle reminder that you're in this together. You did this to her.
And if she's gotta go through nine months of hell to have
a baby, there's no way you're going to sit on the sidelines
and miss out on any of the misery, mister. Go ahead and
practice the line *"We're pregnant."* You've still got a few

months to learn it, since it'll be that long before you'll be allowed to use it in public.

✍ Pregnancy-Test Result Quick Quiz ✍

Your wife is bouncing up and down with joy as a result of a positive pregnancy test. You haven't seen her this happy since…um…well, you've never seen her this happy. Through her hugs and tears of joy she confirms, "I've never been this happy!" Her mom, her sister, her friends—everybody—is going to be so happy for the both of you. You are nine months away from a bouncing new baby. What should you do?

a) Buy a box of good cigars and spread the word.
b) Just make some phone calls. Save the cigars for the actual birth.
c) Bury this away in the secret hidey-hole in your brain right next to the emotional abuse and uncomfortable uncle-touching.

Although answers *a* and *b* sound completely reasonable, the correct answer is *c*. If we've taught you anything, it's that pregnancy is not reasonable.

Silent Partner

The first step after a positive test result is getting your story straight. Universally, women require three months of silence to make sure the pregnancy "sticks." This is especially true if she's had a miscarriage, in which case you'll likely have been on Pregnancy Watch.

Nonetheless, three months of trying to explain why your wife is puking her brains out is good practice for all the lying you'll have to do to your kids for the next twenty years. Like...

- The first time you drank alcohol: "My twenty-first birthday."
- The first time you smoked weed: "Weed? I'm not quite sure what that is."
- The first time you had sex: "Nine months before you were born, and definitely not with a hooker."
- Why it's necessary to know algebra: "Well, it's um... helpful when, uh, you're driving from San Francisco to meet a friend leaving from New York and you, er, want to know what time you'll arrive in Chicago or something."
- Dog gets run over: "He's in doggie heaven because Jesus died so that Superdude would be forgiven for puking on the couch."

Scott had an especially hard time with his wife's ninety-day quiet period. His wife was miserable every single day for three months straight. What's worse is that she was working a few days a week the entire three months. Under normal work circumstances, coworkers wouldn't pry into your personal life too much in front of you; they'd have the courtesy to do it behind your back. But Scott's wife was working for her family's business, which is an altogether different story.

His wife puked several times a day for three months straight. Intuitively recognizing an opportunity to be horrible, the mother-in-law stepped in. "Is everything okay? You don't seem yourself. Did Scott do something he shouldn't have?" Scott's wife politely brushed off her mother's "concerns," telling her that everything was fine.

The mother-in-law decided it was time to go right to the source of her daughter's problems, Scott. "Is everything okay at home?" she asked. (Translation: "If you're doing anything to cause my daughter pain, I will exterminate you.")

"Everything's fine," Scott replied. (Translation: "Your daughter's pregnant. Please don't hurt me.") With just a few threatening and cowering words, they had reached an understanding. Scott spoke little to the mother-in-law for the duration of the pregnancy. In fact, to this day, years after the above incident, they have exchanged only about five hundred words. As Dudes, this is a lesson we can all learn from Scott.

☠ The Mother-in-Law Says ☠

"Shame and guilt are your most valuable resources."

Her Milkshake

The Dudes have some good news and some bad news.

Good news: Here come the juggs! Your wife's melons are going to start growing to a size you've often dreamed about. Her fog lights will begin swelling almost immediately and will continue until they are at least two to three cup sizes larger. She will have a bona fide set of bigguns. Like with the hot chick at work who always wears a v-neck, you will be hard-pressed to look your wife in the eye for months to come. Her love bubbles will be large, supple, firm, beautiful. Her milk cans will be tit-tanic for months and months to come. Be sure to enjoy those bikini stuffers—they will be one of the few joys of the whole process.

Bad news: No touching allowed. There will be a woman with big, beautiful, swollen rib cushions roaming your house and, just like at a strip club, you won't be allowed to touch her sweater meat. And don't expect a private dance in exchange for a $20 in her g-string either. The slightest movements will likely cause her flesh bulbs pain. (Unlike strip clubs, however, you won't have to pay a cover or be forced to buy at least two $8 sodas.)

(**Worse news:** Like the Nile River in flood season, your wife's ample boobies will bring forth fertility and life to an otherwise desolate environment. However, when the river recedes to preflood levels, all will be barren and lifeless. Basically, they will resemble naked Star Jones a year after gastric bypass. Worry not, though. When that happens, and it will, The Dudes will come to your rescue with our newest volume, *The Dudes' Guide to Affordable Plastic Surgery*.)

At the pink, perky epicenter of this subject is the nipple. You wouldn't think there'd be so much ground to cover concerning the nipple, but you're not writing this book, are you? In fact, there is so much ground to cover on the nipple that The Dudes actually considered writing an entirely separate book on the nipple. However, the idea of writing pages and pages of material on nipples seemed overwhelming (heck, we're getting sick of the word *nipple* already), so instead we slapped together this handy nipple chart to help prepare you for the shock of nipple transformation during pregnancy. Basically, as your wife's juggs expand, so will her nipples and surrounding areola. In order to gauge how much your wife's nipples will grow, follow the simple instructions below.

1. Match above *sample nipples* to *actual nipple* (see Figure I).
2. Cut out appropriate *sample nipple*.
3. Hold up to *actual nipple* to attain *reference nipple*.
4. Add three sizes to *reference nipple* to attain *estimate nipple*.

*For full effect, color *estimate nipple* hue of *actual nipple*, and secure *estimate nipple* to *actual nipple* with latex-based adhesive.

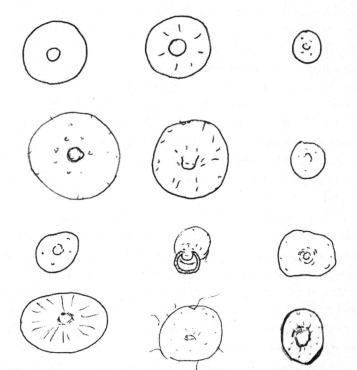

Figure I

The nipples and surrounding flesh mountains can take on a life of their own during pregnancy. As boob transformation continues, expect more updates from The Dudes in forthcoming chapters. As an indication of how important this subject is to us, please note that we just used the word *nipple* twenty-three times (including just now).

Gut Feelings

Although during the first month, your wife's little, parasitic cell mass is only about the size of a pencil eraser or smaller, it is still able to convey the emotion of spite. It does this by making your wife physically, mentally, and emotionally exhausted. She'll be tired all day and unable to sleep at night (it seems that even embryos are amused by irony). And rest assured, she'll be happy to pass along the misery to you. What's more, this will likely continue for the duration of pregnancy, only to be replaced afterward by fatigue and sleeplessness for an entirely different reason.

Food cravings also begin in the first month of pregnancy— not the storied *pickles and ice cream* variety, but the *I have to eat right now* variety. The cravings come out of nowhere and can cause dizziness and nausea, but mostly they cause stomach pain that can only be cured by your wife shoving anything that is remotely edible down her throat. You may want to encourage your wife to carry snacks with her in her car or purse: believe us when we tell you that you don't want to be stuck in the car with her during the onslaught of one of these attacks.

Interestingly, Bill and his wife were in the dark about this type of craving for the first several weeks of their pregnancy. Then one night during these first weeks, Bill was bitching his way through his seventh viewing of his *Lord of the Rings: The Fellowship of the Ring* DVD, which had been released the day before. And while he was yelling at the screen, saying "This is supposed to be Middle Earth? You can totally see a car driving in the background!" he noticed his wife get up and run into the kitchen.

Doubled over in pain, she was able to yell out in a voice that wasn't hers, "Get me some fucking food now." Like a brave yet reluctant young hobbit, Bill-bo knew that he must save the elven Aerosmith princess from imminent danger. With the fiery Eye of Sauron watching his every move, he knew his quest would be wrought with peril and temptation.

Bill-bo's large, hairy feet swiftly carried him to the pantry, where he spotted the most wondrous of snack foods, an unopened bag of Funyuns. While simultaneously rushing the crunchy, oniony rings to the imperiled maiden and opening the bag, Bill-bo stopped in his tracks. He was overwhelmed with temptation.

> *One ring to rule them all*
> *One ring to feed them*
> *One ring to bring them all*
> *And in the darkness eat them*
> *In the kitchen pantry where the Funyuns lie.*

"Thieves! They're filthy little thieves. My Precious. Curse them, we hates them! The Funyuns ours it is, and we wants it."

"Where's my goddamn food?!?" Bill's wife shrieked as Bill-bo snapped out of his snack-induced trance in time to feed the angry princess and savor some wonderful Funyuns for himself. For now, he would remain lord of the onion rings, at least until their splendor made him jealous and miserable with gas.

Dr. Dude Says

"Be sure to eat a variety of foods during pregnancy. Nutrients and calories are vital to a growing baby and mother, so try to save some food for your wife as well."

Scent of a Woman

In addition to her exciting new hunger pangs and yelling proficiency, your wife will inevitably develop an acute sense of smell. But her new bloodhoundlike olfactory abilities will only irritate her. Basically, she'll become a bloated, nauseous superhero with the lamest superpower of all time. Like Aquaman with a fish allergy, her new powers will only serve to torment her while she develops aversions to the odors of certain foods or even to nonfood odors. For example, meat and/or Windex are just two more items on a growing list of things that can induce vomiting during pregnancy, a list that may include the following:

1. Garbage
2. Body odor
3. Leftovers in the fridge
4. Coffee
5. Gasoline
6. Hand lotion
7. Air
8. You

What's more, she will probably become nauseated by simply *thinking* about any of the above-mentioned items. Scott's wife actually used to become ill just imagining the smell of her grandmother's basement, the basement of a house which, by the way, was bulldozed and replaced by a minimart in the mid-1980s. What we're saying here is insanely significant: Scott's wife got sick from a smell that hasn't existed on this planet for twenty-plus years. If that's not mind-boggling, we don't know what is.

What sounds like a modest inconvenience can easily become a major issue for some couples. Case in point: our friend Tony. Tony had just returned from a long day of shaking down local small-business owners to find a half-cooked manicotti dinner on the stove and his newly pregnant wife, Carmella, cowering in the basement, muttering to herself, "That smell. That awful smell." After getting her to calm down, Tony suggested they go upstairs and talk about it. "No. I can't go up there. The smell is up there." She wouldn't budge.

"What-ah smell-ah?" Tony asked in his thick Italian accent. All he could smell was the sweet, spicy aroma of his wife's homemade marinara sauce cooking on the stove. Realizing what was happening, Tony slapped his head saying, "Mamma mia!" further reinforcing stereotypes. While preparing a big, Sicilian dinner, Carmella discovered she was sickened by the odor of marinara sauce. And with the highest of Italian holidays just a week away, the family would be gathering to feast on marinara-soaked pasta, sausage, spumoni, etc. Tony knew this would be the worst Columbus Day ever.

Every holiday for the duration of Carmella's pregnancy proved to be a challenge. Tony and the kids, Anthony Jr.

and Autumn, would be happily feasting in the dining room while Carmella and her Caesar salad commiserated on the back porch. Carmella would eventually lose her fear of red sauce, but things were never really the same again.

Of course, this is just the beginning. Yes, your wife's brain has begun its battle with your wife's body. The result is kind of like knocking back a few sleeping pills and speed with a shot of NyQuil and a Red Bull chaser and seeing what happens. The Dudes recommend against this, though, as does the estate of Elvis Presley.

Coitus Interruptus

With all the robo-fucking you've been doing for the past several months, you may have grown accustomed to it. And though it may have become lifeless and vanilla, it beats the alternative of paying for sex. But as sure as you could count on nightly porking leading up to conception, you can count on it stopping almost immediately after your wife becomes pregnant (so much for weaning).

Don't be surprised if your wife imposes a four- to six-week sexual moratorium. In which case The Dudes suggest you take this early-pregnancy dry spell to start making deposits in your internal "spank bank." The spank bank is the area of your brain reserved for "depositing" dirty images that you can conjure up at a later time—or "withdraw"—to help you through the many autoerotic episodes you'll experience for the next nine to twenty-four months. Congratulations, your new account with Spank of America is now open. (If it's any consolation, the symptoms of pregnancy—including but not limited to fatigue, bloating, headache, dizziness, absent-mindedness, and spite—usually make for an uncomfortable roll in the sack anyway. More on that later.)

Bad Head

If you're anything like every guy who's ever gotten a girl knocked up, there are certain aspects of pregnancy that will creep up on your brain and kick your brain's ass without even a hint of mercy. This will often happen shortly after you find out that she's pregnant.

At first, when you hear that she's going to be having your baby, you might be the happiest guy in the world. You'll imagine yourself playing catch with the boy, or doing some other stereotypical thing you do with a girl. But as The Dudes have discovered, that happiness can quickly turn into fear and paranoia as you begin to slip uncomfortably back into reality.

As your brain gets used to the idea of your wife being pregnant, you will start to look at the world differently. It's not just you anymore—it's you and her and the baby. You've entered into a whole new realm of responsibility that you can't really appreciate until it settles in. Your brain will commence asking you a series of rhetorical questions that you'll irrationally try to answer. And who wants to answer a bunch of rhetorical questions?

You might start to resent and/or envy people who lead the carefree, childless life that you just cast aside. "How dare they not have to worry about supporting a child?" you might angrily ask yourself. That will inevitably be followed with "Holy shit, what the fuck was I thinking? I'm not ready for this!"

It gets better (worse), because those thoughts are always followed by more gut-wrenching what-if's.

■ What if I lose my job?
■ What if we have only one income?
■ What if the baby is born with four asses?

Something Scott's wife found particularly annoying was his propensity to monitor every chemical that she came into contact with. He checked and rechecked food labels. He did Internet searches. And even more annoying were his much-too-vivid descriptions of what awful things said chemicals could do to an unborn child (e.g., four asses).

Thoughts like these are common, and The Dudes sympathize. Unfortunately, while we may sympathize, there's pretty much nothing we can do to help. You can either wait and hope that these thoughts run their course and go away, or you can do what we do and bury them deep down inside so we can get back to thinking about sex again.

Dudes in Cubes

The extent of the pregnancy knowledge possessed by most guys with no kids usually comes down to this: women eat all the time and get huge. So when you start out on your beautiful and wholly fulfilling journey to fatherhood, it's a good idea, from time to time, to ask your peers for advice. Dudes you know who have been there before tend to view the world a little differently than you do. And they can often provide you with invaluable advice on how to deal with the various "joys" of pregnancy. Sometimes their advice will apply directly to your situation, and sometimes they'll laugh and make fun of you for asking such stupid questions.

Scott had only to look over his standard (soul-crushing) 4-foot-high cubicle walls at work to find several guys who had either been there before or had no clue what a woman was. They would readily, and often without provocation, offer up bits of wisdom. Some bits of wisdom would relate directly to pregnancy, while other bits would relate directly to whoever the asshole was who fucked up the printer again. We promise to share with you as much of this pregnancy wisdom as we can in order to help you through the months ahead.

The Dudes firmly believe that stereotyping is Science's most valuable social organization tool. Given that, we try to use it as often as possible to take the guesswork out of daily life. The workplace is the perfect place to use this valuable tool. Over the months of pregnancy, Scott came to refer to the advice-giving work people as The Dudes In Cubes, or DICs. For easier reference, he further divided them into three even more precise generalizations.

Bitter Divorce Guy

First, every dude knows the guy who's been there before, the guy who got married young, usually because he accidentally got his girlfriend pregnant. The marriage was rocky from the start, and they tried to patch things up by having another kid. Everyone knows that nothing fixes a troubled marriage like a second kid. Add a little "minor" infidelity to the mix, along with dash of a superiority complex, and the result is the guy Scott's dubbed Bitter Divorce Guy.

Bitter Divorce Guy's advice is almost always some variation of "Dude, don't ever get married; it fucking sucks" or "Dude, I ain't never getting married again, that's for goddamn sure." We're not really sure if the second one qualifies as advice, but if you hear it enough, it starts to sound reasonable. He repeatedly gave Scott this "advice" knowing full well that Scott was already happily married. Bitter Divorce Guy's horrible experience almost always serves as an ego boost for Scott and a veritable road map on how to destroy a marriage. However, there are occasional pearls of wisdom that can be gained from Bitter Divorce Guy.

Sensitive Guy

Sometimes it's important to keep a journal of your feelings. It can help you cope with the stresses and pressures of being a father-to-be. It can also help you better understand the complex emotions and feelings that your partner is going through. On top of that, it will provide great reading material years down the road. It will allow you and your partner to experience the joys of pregnancy all over again, while looking at pictures of your beautiful baby's birth.

That's the kind of ridiculous crap that Scott heard from Sensitive Guy.

The Dudes know you might find it difficult to take pregnancy advice from a guy who thinks the rhythm method (aka "Nature's condom") is a viable form of contraception, but don't be so quick to judge. You can bet that a guy with three kids and four on the way will definitely have some quality pregnancy advice to offer. While trying his hardest not to sound too preachy in the office, Sensitive Guy would periodically relate feminine-sounding pregnancy advice to Scott during work hours.

Foreign Guy

As far as we know, pregnancy works pretty much the same in every country. Sure, every culture has its own customs and practices, but The Dudes tend to stick with what we know.

That doesn't necessarily mean that we aren't open to suggestions from someone whose country confuses and frightens us; it just means we're closed-minded and shallow.

Scott would always take a break from work to listen to whatever pearls of wisdom Foreign Guy had to offer. Sometimes Foreign Guy would rail on and on about the lack of seafood diversity in this country, and sometimes he'd praise the high quality of programming offered by cable television. It was impossible for Scott to tell from day to day what Foreign Guy was going to say. So it was usually worthwhile to work past the thick accent to find the gems.

Scott was sitting around the office one day, talking to some of the guys, when he mentioned that he and his wife were contemplating trying to have kids. He didn't really think about how the DICs would react before he brought it up, but that was before he'd properly stereotyped them.

Before most of the other guys could really say anything, Bitter Divorce Guy was working himself up into a concerned frenzy. "Dude, Scott, kids are great and all, but you've gotta think about where this whole marriage thing leads. Seriously, man, trying to get her pregnant is fun and all, but it's all downhill from there. I ain't never getting married again, I can tell ya that much right now. They should outlaw marriage in Congress. End of story."

Hearing this tirade from Bitter Divorce Guy, Sensitive Guy proudly proclaimed that he had been married for fourteen of the best, most wonderful years of his life. He couldn't understand why Bitter Divorce Guy was so upset and suggested that if Bitter Divorce Guy had been more in touch with his wife's feelings and needs, maybe he wouldn't be bitter and divorced.

As Sensitive Guy was suggesting to Scott that he start writing a pregnancy journal like he did, Bitter Divorce Guy interrupted and told Scott that Sensitive Guy's wife was probably cheating on him. He then told Sensitive Guy to write about *that* in his "new-age wuss journal" and stormed off.

Foreign Guy didn't really want to get involved in the commotion, but he pulled Scott aside later on. He told Scott that his mom knew the "secrets of producing the male child," and that he'd arrange for his mom to call Scott later that week. Foreign Guy said that his mom had already had two boys, so she knew what she was talking about. Scott laughed at the notion of talking to Foreign Mom and quickly forgot the whole episode.

The following night, Scott's phone rang, and his caller ID displayed a string of consonants the likes of which have rarely been seen. Imagine his surprise when he picked up the phone only to hear Foreign Guy carrying on on the other end. Scott confusedly asked Foreign Guy how he got his phone number but was ignored, as Foreign Guy was busy conferencing Foreign Mom into the conversation, live from the old country. Because of the time change, Scott figured that wherever she was, it must be very early in the morning sometime in the middle of next week. Foreign Mom started speaking loudly and foreignly in her native tongue, whatever the hell that was. Foreign Guy had to translate for Scott all the uncomfortable sex details his mother was describing unashamedly. In the end, all Scott got from the call from Foreign Guy's mom (aside from being totally creeped out) was that in order to have a boy, you needed 7 meters of braided rope, some sort of sturdy pulley mechanism, and the magic smoke.

One of the many things you'll have to deal with as a father-to-be is the myriad of pregnancy advice from just about everywhere. While The Dudes will always give it to you straight in this guide, we certainly can't control what the people around you will say. Most of their advice will be harmless and easy to ignore. Some of it, though, will keep you up at night, worried that your unborn baby's head will spontaneously combust at random or some other horribleness. When hearing such advice, keep in mind that it's almost always well intentioned. As in, the road to hell is paved with it. Thus, simply smile, nod, and filter out the bits you think you can use.

Not So Bad, Eh?

The friction burns on your wiener have healed. You've successfully navigated the pregnancy test without getting pee on you. You told the right people—no one—the news. Your wife weathered a few weeks of morning sickness. Now you may be thinking, "Hey, this might not be so bad!" Really? That's kind of like saying

- "Condom, schmondom! Herpes died out with the 1970s!"
- "I think this L. Ron Hubbard book could really help me get my life in order!"

or

- "I'm such a stupid dumbass, I can't believe how stupid and dumb I am. God, I'm stupid!"

You get the idea. You've only made it through chapter 1. And although this is probably the most you've read that doesn't affect your GPA or allow you to choose your own adventure (yet), you've still got a few pages to go.

Myth vs. Fact

Myth: Pregnancy makes marital bonds stronger than ever.
Fact: Pregnancy makes your wife's boobs bigger than ever.

Myth: Frequent urination is a negative side effect of pregnancy.
Fact: Frequent urination is the least of your problems.

Myth: Pregnancy tests are accurate and affordable.
Fact: Pregnancy-test purchases can seriously cut into your beer money.

Myth: The Church of Scientology has changed the lives of thousands for the better.
Fact: Lawyers from the church of Scientology have assured us the above myth is accurate.

Myth: Your wife's enlarged breasts may be sensitive to touch.
Fact: Your enlarged unit will be sensitive to touch.

CHAPTER TWO

Weeks 5–9

The second month of pregnancy offers a lovely bouquet of new experiences while generously holding over all the lovely experiences of month one. Bloating, dizziness, fatigue, sleeplessness, and now gas problems all become part of the daily routine. And it's even possible that your wife will experience some of these symptoms.

What a Waist

The topic of your wife's changing body will be a touchy area for her during her pregnancy. Fear not, however. Your wife will *not* gain 35 to 50 pounds during her pregnancy. She will *not* eat everything she can get her grubby, life-giving hands on. She will *not* get painful stomach cramps at a moment's notice and scream at you to get her some "motherfucking food" immediately. She will *not* crave unusual food items like blueberry bagels with mustard, spicy foreign sausage, artichoke dip (for breakfast), pizza with Catalina dressing, Froot Loops on cookie dough ice cream, etc. Note: She will *not* be upset when there aren't enough sprinkles on her Krispy Kreme donuts. She will *not* be upset about her weight gain.

Time for a Dude's Guide
Choose-Your-Own-Destiny Adventure!

If you totally buy the previous statements, turn to the following page and continue reading!

If you think The Dudes may be pulling a fast one on you, turn to page 40 now!

Hahahahahaha! Oh, man. That's so funny. We can't *believe* you bought that. Oh, man...hang on a sec. We've gotta catch our breath. Whew! Good times.

The Dudes are firm believers in sarcasm and the valuable lessons it can teach. *Note: The previous sentence was not sarcastic. (Neither was that sentence).* So if your brain can figure out how to turn the page without forgetting to make you breathe, please continue.

Ahhhh, you have chosen wisely. I guess all those years of strategizing your neutral-good fighter's destiny through the dungeon master's realm have really paid off for you in the long run, nerdo.

If all is going according to plan, your wife isn't even showing yet. That's fantastic, and we highly recommend you step back and take it all in. Yes, take a good long—last—look at the woman you married. Go ahead—take as much time as you need. We'll wait. You might even want to have sex if you can swing it. What the hell, take some pictures if you can get away with it—anything you need to do to remember her just the way she is. Like a horde of angry zombies at an all-you-can-eat brains buffet, things are about to get messy.

Babies tend to destroy a woman's body from the inside out. Literally. It's not quite as dramatic as the movie *Alien,* where the creepy little parasite alien popped right out of that guy's stomach, but the parallels are painfully relevant. Your wife's uterus is normally the size of a fist. At full term, it will be approximately the size, shape, and consistency of an automatic transmission. This will rearrange her inner organs, smashing them up against her bladder and making it difficult for her diaphragm to do its job of making your wife breathe. You'll be living with a large woman who can't breathe and constantly has to pee. Is that on the list of traits you look for in a woman when you're sober? No.

Not So Fun Fact

Science tells us that your wife's uterus will have become
more than five hundred times its original size by the
time she goes into labor...kind of like his morning boner.
Thanks for the perspective, Science.

Beforemath and Aftermath

After reading the above, you might be wondering if your
wife will ever return to her Pre-Pregnancy Hotness. This
question is an extremely important one to The Dudes, and
it actually has three possible answers: no, never, and maybe
[Figure II]. We'll examine them in that order.

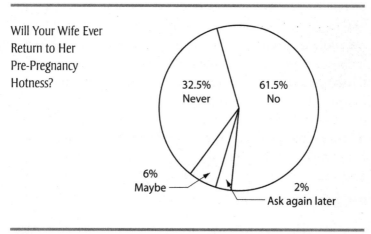

Will Your Wife Ever
Return to Her
Pre-Pregnancy
Hotness?

32.5%
Never

61.5%
No

6%
Maybe

2%
Ask again later

Figure II

No.

Sorry, dude, but it just won't happen. Welcome to the majority. While it might be possible to regain part of it, there's a good chance that it's gone forever. We sincerely hope you took some good pictures. We also sincerely hope that you sent them to us. Seriously.

Call it genetics, call it fate, call it the great hidden camera show of the gods, but when it's all said and done, the results are still the same: your wife's body will be forever altered by pregnancy, and only on the rarest of rare occasions is this a good thing. In the end, her hips will be wider, her tits will deflate (they'll get even smaller than they were before), and she might even be left with purplish stretch marks all over her stomach. Don't worry about that, though, because those purple stretch marks will eventually turn white and never go away. Ever.

The Dudes are constantly in awe of how much Nature hates us. There is some hope here, though: if your wife can get motivated enough to eat properly and exercise regularly, she can return to about 80 percent of her prepregnancy hotness. If she exercises *during* pregnancy, the percentage rises to 90 percent. It'll probably be up to you to motivate her, though. Our wise friend Dave once told us that you can't make a fat girl skinny by not calling her fat. He's twice divorced, but we still consider him wise.

Never.

Our friend Science tells us that younger women have a much greater potential for Post-Pregnancy Hotness Recovery than older women. The Post-Pregnancy Hotness Recovery Factor Ψ can be attained by using the following formula:

$$\psi = 0 \text{x(B)} \sum_{n=0}^{\infty} \frac{G + 1.0042}{c^\wedge n}$$

where *B* is her bra size (in hexadecimal), *G* is the gravitational constant, *c* is the speed of light, and *n* is her age as it approaches infinity.

As Ψ approaches zero, a full recovery is assured. You can rest uneasily assured, however, that Science tells us a zero factor is mathematically, and thus practically, impossible. Again, thanks a lot, Science.

That's why it cracks The Dudes up to see people waiting till they're thirty-four and "ready" to have kids. Being "ready" to have kids is one of the biggest jokes in the history of modern thirtysomething society, along with the following:

- Accessorize with a designer dog.
- Wheatgrass smoothies will make you not fat.
- You look totally awesome driving that hybrid.
- Professional soccer is exciting, and you look cool in your Beckham jersey.

Really, what the holy crap are you waiting for? More money? Stability? Hell, children rob you of these things anyway, so you might as well start early.

As you can see from the above formula, after a certain age, it just won't happen. No matter what she claims to try, the postpartum pounds, among other things, are locked permanently in place. The brutal, dimpled irony is that Nature doesn't tell you what the drop-dead target age is. There is no convenient age stamp on the bottom of her foot that says "Have children before age thirty-four." It's all guesswork after thirty, and the longer you wait, the more likely your gamble will not pay off.

So, to the guy who thinks it's a good idea to wait to have kids, The Dudes think you're taking an unnecessary risk with little or no payoff at the end. Sure, you get to go out a few more times each month because you don't have to worry about kids, but in the grand scheme of things, is that really worth it? We say no f'ing way. Even if you think you've got the system beat by having enough money to hire your wife a personal trainer, you'll still lose. She'll most likely start banging the trainer and take half your money anyway. We've seen it happen. To Dave.

Maybe.

There are two hotness categories of Maybe, Lucky Hotness and the wonderful outcome of something The Dudes like to call The Metamorphosis.

The first is the group of women who are lucky enough to actually have pregnancy make them look *hotter* than they were *before* getting themselves knocked up. We know how insane that can sound to most dudes, but Science tells us it's possible, and he's almost never wrong. Incredibly, Lucky Hotness will sometimes happen to women who are naturally skinny to begin with. Pregnancy can give them a decent figure entirely by accident. It's sorta like Pregnancy fell asleep at the wheel, veered off the road, hit a tree, and turned into a big pile of ten-dollar bills. If you happen to be married to a woman like this, congratulations. As an interesting social experiment, you might have fun trying to keep track of how many dudes stare at your wife's brand-new ass a year after she's given birth. You can bet we'll be staring.

The second Maybe category is something so spectacular that its manifestation must actually be seen to be believed. We call it The Metamorphosis. It's that magical point sometime after childbirth when your wife sheds her awkward, pear-shaped pregnancy cocoon and emerges as a Mom I'd Like to Fuck, or a MILF.

No one knows quite how this happens. Modern medicine has spent millions of dollars earmarked for cancer research trying to explain it. If you're one of the lucky ones, this logic-defying transformation will happen to your wife. You'll be the envy of all your friends and neighbors. You'll have survived pregnancy and emerged triumphantly on the other side, baby in one hand and your wife's sweet, sweet ass in the other. The idea of the MILF is so fascinating that we will further explore this miracle of pregnancy in greater detail in a later chapter. For now, we'll just say that in day-to-day life, MILFs are granted more leniency than ordinary hot chicks as far as what passes for hot. They are hot because they are MILFs and are MILFs because they are hot. We told you this was complicated. Amazingly, that apparent paradox doesn't seem to matter to dudes. Consequently, MILFs get much more attention. This is much to the irritation of the above-mentioned ordinary hot chick who, consequently, has to work that much harder to get noticed when there's a MILF around.

Having a hot MILF at your side is a badge of honor, but unfortunately there is really no way of knowing if The Metamorphosis will take place for your wife *before* you get her pregnant. You just have to pray hard that Science will somehow come to your rescue. Good luck.

There's No *U* in Dignity

Pregnant women go through so many changes that you will often find yourself questioning your will to live. There is no way to escape this. No way to cure it. There is no supplement or quick fix of any kind. The girl you once knew will be forever changed by pregnancy and motherhood. This is not so much bad as it is different. It will, however, become bad if you do not learn to properly deal with it sooner rather than later. Like some sort of ninja marine, you must learn to adapt and overcome. It will do you no good whatsoever to do battle with her while she's pregnant.

We know, however, that from time to time you will not be able to resist arguing over something you consider too absurd to be ignored. Maybe it's her overwhelming fear that you've lost your ability to drive a car, or the worries that you'll end up in a ball of flames the next time you go to the store. It could be any number of horrible scenarios involving your demise, your insensitivity, or your lack of enthusiasm in tending to her needs. But whatever it is, it is best to simply *avoid the argument*. The Dudes' tried-and-true concept of avoiding the argument is the cornerstone of any and all advice that we offer and is the basis for any Dudes-approved relationship. It applies to many circumstances, pregnancy or otherwise.

The concept of avoiding the argument dates back to ancient Greece, when a Greek guy decided to avoid arguing with his wife. As the legend goes, the man, Testiclees, found that when he nodded and agreed (i.e., avoided arguing) with his wife, Labius, he had more time to hang out at the local bathhouse with his friends, Scrotus and Pecticlees. He began cleaning up in his fantasy gladiator league. He quickly became the proud, naked king of the steam room. While The Dudes hardly endorse Testiclees' intentions, his methods started a new era in understanding, or at least dealing with, women.

This knowledge is most important in a pregnancy situation. There is little point in arguing with your wife when her hormone levels are through the roof and you're questioning her sanity. Simply agree with whatever she says, go make her a goddamn sandwich, and keep your smart-ass comments to yourself. There is no pride in pregnancy. Actually, there's no dignity either, but you should have already figured that out by now.

One thing that's very important to remember is that although it may seem otherwise at the time, she will not be pregnant forever. Sure it's great to have some sarcastic fun at your pregnant wife's expense here and there. Saying things like "It's all part of the miracle" or "Better you than me" might make *you* laugh, but they will be remembered. In fact, most of the things that you forget about in two seconds she will remember forever. And payback is hell. So unless you enjoy listening to her telling her mother/sister/girlfriend about what an asshole you were, you need to play your cards right during pregnancy.

☠ **The Mother-in-Law Says** ☠

"Never go to bed angry. Stay up and fight."

[Sigh] "Yes, Dear"

During the next nine months, and even for a few months after the baby arrives, your wife will be prone to extreme mood swings, which seem to somehow be designed to confuse and disorient you. As long as you realize this, these mood extremes are usually easy to detect before they strike and somewhat easier to avoid/escape.

The larger your wife gets, the more insecure she will become. This insecurity will manifest itself in a variety of ways, all of which will be unpleasant for you. Sometimes she'll ask if she's getting fat. Sometimes she'll "need" to spend a great deal of money on new "cute" maternity clothes (clothes, we might add, that she'll only be wearing for a handful of months at most). Sometimes she'll take her childhood doll, dress it up, and head to the baby megastore, where she'll spend hours putting it into various car seats and strollers just to work out the right color scheme. The worst part is that she'll insist that you go with her so you can give her your opinion—an opinion, we might add, that will mean absolutely nothing unless it's the same as hers. Spending hours in the baby megastore sounds exactly like not watching football, which bothers The Dudes greatly.

During episodes like these, it's best to just nod, agree or disagree as appropriate, and find some important reason to go into the garage for an hour or two. The problem will usually resolve itself during your time away. We haven't yet figured out how this resolution works, and there is no way in hell we're sticking around to find out. Maybe Science will give us some answers some day, but we won't hold our breath.

The Toast Incident

Our friend Steve recently told us of an incident that is pretty much a metaphor for all of pregnancy. After a long, exhausting day of working for the man, Steve came home to find his wife even more surly and irritable than usual. Deciding to avoid the inevitable argument (good call, Steve), he slipped into the kitchen to fix himself some dinner. Out of the corner of his eye, he noticed an object on the floor of the living room. Further investigation revealed the object to be a piece of toast with one small bite missing. What follows is the actual conversation that ensued:

Steve: "What's this?"
Wife: "It's toast."
Steve: "Why is it on the floor?"
Wife: "Because I threw it there."
Steve: "Why?"
Wife: "Because I didn't want it."
Steve: "Why didn't you want it??"
Wife: "Because it smelled like toast."

Because it smelled like toast . . . Read that again until the reality of it sinks in. *Because it smelled like toast.* . . . It is with great confidence that The Dudes can say all pregnancies involve many pieces of toast. Your own personal toast could be listening to her complain about morning sickness, listening to her complain about swollen ankles, or listening to her complain about weight gain. In this case, Steve's toast just happened to be an actual piece of toast. But it was only one small piece of toasted bread that was part of the all-encompassing, crusty loaf that is pregnancy.

✐ Avoiding the Argument Quick Quiz ✐

Our Latino friend Jesus' wife is about five months pregnant and is convinced that he's cheating on her. They battle back and forth about his alleged cheating for hours. What should Jesus do?

a) Fight for his good name. He's not cheating. He shouldn't have to listen to these ridiculous accusations.
b) Cheat. He's already got his scarlet *A*. It's his predetermined destiny.
c) Avoid the argument. Go play video games. Eat some chicken wings.

While *a* and *b* may be your knee-jerk answers, you're wrong. We do sympathize, though. Oddly enough, *c* is actually the correct answer. Although *c* may not feel right, it is the only option that allows for video games and tasty chicken wings. That's what Jesus would do.

Big Girls Do Cry

Sometimes, your pregnant wife will burst into tears for no apparent (to you) reason. It could be that she's watching one of those baby shows on TV, or maybe she just saw a little kid walk past on the sidewalk. It's hard to tell. The most bizarre tears, however, are those that even *she* can't explain.

It's strange, and sometimes funny, to watch your wife burst into tears without so much as a word from you. Knowing full well that she's crying for no reason, she still can't stop it. For example, our neighbor Tom was watching television one evening when his mother-in-law called. He said hello, then handed the phone over to his pregnant wife. After talking for about forty-five seconds, his wife suddenly broke down and started to cry. Usually that meant that she and her mother were talking about what an asshole he was. That evening, however, he didn't recall actually doing anything wrong. His wife had been fine one minute earlier, so he felt safe to ask her what was wrong when she got off the phone. She went on to say that her mom had been describing an outfit she'd gotten earlier that day, and that her mom's description was so cute that she couldn't help but cry. Tom shook his head in disbelief and went back to watching television. Thus making his wife cry again.

Our friend Jack told us of a similar incident that happened to him. His pregnant wife had been out shopping all day while he was home working in the yard. When she returned from the mall, she waved, smiled, and took her bags into the house. About a half hour later, Jack finished up in the yard and went inside. His wife was nowhere to be found. Getting a little worried, he called out her name. Nothing. He listened...the faint sound of sobbing could be heard coming from kitchen pantry. Worried, he carefully opened the door. Peeking inside, he found his wife leaning against the shelf with tears streaming down her face. She had a half-eaten bag of M&M's in one hand and a brand-new picture frame in the other.

Jack gently nudged his wife out of the pantry and sat her down at the kitchen table. She had almost stopped crying at that point, so he asked her what was wrong. Still holding the M&M's and picture frame, she started crying again and showed him the picture frame. "Look," she said. "Look at that." Jack looked at the frame, but it was shrink-wrapped, and she hadn't put a picture in it yet. He had no idea what she was getting at, and he handed it back to her. "See what I mean," she said. Jack, still having no idea what she was talking about, simply said "Yes," gave her a hug, and went back out to the garage.

Jack later found out what she'd been crying about. Apparently, the random picture of a happy family that was in the new picture frame when his wife bought it was the cause of her tears. In the picture, the woman was holding a baby. That was it. That picture of an anonymous family had triggered an M&M binge and about twenty minutes of tears. The Dudes still haven't come up with an appropriate response to situations like this. It's best just to adopt a sympathetic look, nod knowingly, and tell them that everything will be all right.

Helpful Advice

In extreme cases, the mood swings of a pregnant woman can mimic those of a clinically diagnosed manic-depressive. The Dudes suggest that you find a clever way of dealing with that. Somehow.

Silent Butt Deadly

The biology involved with a woman's pregnancy is mind-boggling. Did you know the placenta can create any anatomical hormone except luteinizing hormone? Did you know that during gestation a woman's blood is never mixed with that of her fetus? Most importantly, did you know a woman can actually fart more than you during her pregnancy? It's a little-known fact, but her trouser coughs will put your butt burps to shame. If your wife is anything like every woman on the planet, in a group setting, she will politely excuse herself to excuse herself elsewhere. But when she gets you alone, it's a ten-year-old boys' sleepover all over again.

The interesting ones are the sleepfarts. The Dudes have heard that they can last upwards of five seconds. Go ahead and make a farting noise for five whole seconds. See? Again…shocking. If you're having trouble sleeping, you can count your wife's sleepfarts instead of sheep. You should be able to nod off after thirty or so (of course, the high methane content in the air may have something to do with the drowsiness).

We suggest accepting her air biscuits as a throwing down of the gaseous gauntlet. Make a game out of it. Don't be surprised if you're easily defeated in both the duration *and* odor categories. Yes, it'll be like poker night for nine straight months at your house. By the time the baby arrives, you may feel shame about your shortcomings but proud of your wife at the same time.

Aural Exam Too

At around the six-week mark, your wife's doctor will want to get a look at the tiny embryo that calls your wife's guts home. It may seem obvious that the easiest way to get a look at your pea-sized child-to-be would be to shrink down to the size of, say, a huge penis, and jam yourself uncomfortably into her birthhole until you get close enough to have a first-person look-see for yourself. We're guessing that the dude who invented the ultrasound thought this very thing, but then got hung up on lighting issues. Nonetheless, he fashioned some sort of medieval curling iron–type instrument to do the dirty work, and the vaginal ultrasound was born.

We say with complete sincerity that all dudes actually believe that women love trips to their gynecologists because they get to have instruments inserted into them. "If I were a girl, I'd love it," we all think in that situation. Your nodding while reading this just confirms that. However, we've been told that a percentage of women (must be a small one) actually find the experience disconcerting. Nonetheless, your wife is likely to have the time of her life when the ultrasound technician lubes up and inserts the business end and points out a blip on the grainy screen purported to be your kid that will be born on this specific date. Plus, your wife's awkward clean-up after the procedure will help remind you of the sweaty night that your little grainy blip was conceived.

Seriously, What About Me?

As you experience the trials and tribulations of pregnancy, you may be selflessly thinking, "Will my wife ever really understand what I'm going through?" The Dudes can confidently answer, "No, she can't." For example, you'll most likely want to celebrate the impregnation of your wife by buying a brand-new, kick-ass 50-inch flat-panel high-definition plasma television (with wall-mount swivel bracket). She'll understand that about as much as you'll understand her need to constantly spend your kick-ass TV money on prenatal vitamins. Have you noticed how expensive those things are? Well, you sure as hell will when your precious TV money is being squandered on them.

Other questions on your deeply troubled mind may be

1. Can we afford this?
2. Will the baby be healthy?
3. How much is this going to cost me?
4. Will the baby love me?
5. Will I love the baby?
6. Seriously, how much are we talkin' here?
7. Will a second job be necessary, and if so, how many extra hours can my wife work?

The Dudes understand that a variety of very important questions are haunting you. Rest assured that we will do our best to answer them in great detail while interjecting our own awesome opinions along the way. Plus, if we can't answer them, we'll do our best to distract you from that fact by making up top-10 lists and talking about boobies.

But before we really get into answering your questions, there's one thing we feel we should just get out of the way right up front, and that's to answer the question that you forgot to ask: question 8. What will happen to my collection of nice things? We're your friends, after all, and when brutal honesty is needed, we're here to deliver. So, let's get started with question 8.

As dudes, one of our favorite pastimes is the acquisition of things. Whether it's your golf clubs, your collection of vintage WWF wrestling figures with wrestling ring and steel cage, or an autographed box of Mr. T cereal, we take pride in our nice collections. We recommend that sometime before your child is born, you gather up all the nice things you own, put them in a big pile in your garage, and systematically destroy the shit out of them. Please, for us, find the joy in it. It's there. This might not make sense to you right now, but you have to trust us on this. The idea of *you* having the distinct pleasure of breaking all *your* cool shit before your kid gets a chance to do it is strangely rewarding. The destruction will happen regardless, and why should some kid who you hardly even know get to have all the fun?

Account Ability

Money is probably one of your biggest concerns at this point. As well it should be, because a typical problem-free birth will run you about $6,000. The cost increases exponentially if there are any procedures requiring special care, such as the dreaded episiotomy, aka "The Big Snip," or the dreaded C-section, aka "The Big Scar." It's not unheard-of to cost as much as $30,000 or more for a delivery in these extreme cases. Our estimates don't even include the nine months of prenatal office visits at $250 bucks a pop or the steadily increasing grocery bill. We sincerely hope you had your insurance premiums paid up when you got her knocked up.

If that's the case, then you can rest assured that your basic working-stiff health insurance will significantly soften the financial blow. On the other hand, if you're still on the high school football team, you'll have to put in some extra hours making cones at Dairy Queen to help your parents cover the costs.

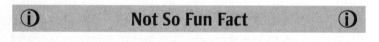

ⓘ   **Not So Fun Fact**   ⓘ

Most insurance plans consider pregnancy
to be a sickness. The Dudes also consider
pregnancy to be a sickness.

Make sure you know what's covered by your insurance plan and what isn't. That way you'll know exactly what to expect when the hospital billing statements start arriving. In fact, some statements might actually arrive before you even start to *think* about the delivery. Some hospitals make you pay your deductible as far in advance as possible so that the bean counters can be assured that they'll get their full cut of the blood money later, when you're too busy with the baby to answer those calls from the collection agency.

Fun Experiment

After your child is born, ask the hospital for the itemized bill. They usually don't itemize unless you specifically ask them to. You'll be amazed at how much that catheter actually cost.

It's almost impossible to predict what this baby's going to cost you, since the bills will be so spread out. And aside from the pregnancy and birth, you should probably look down the road as well. For example, if it's a girl, she's going to need a pony or something. If it's a boy, he's going to need a new bowling ball with his initials on it—initials that might, if carefully selected ahead of time, happen to be the same as yours.

Money Shot

The Dudes think we've found the answer to child financial planning, though, and our plan is truly groundbreaking in its simplicity. All you have to do is start thinking of your child as a monthly payment, and try to get yourself used to the idea.

We know that at first it might sound "mean" and "selfish" to think that way, but trust us, you won't love the kid any less because of it. In fact, we think you'll soon be thanking us for revolutionizing the way your baby is viewed in the eyes of your dwindling bank account. Simply insert this new payment into the existing bill-paying cycle, and watch as your money works for you. And then there's reality…

Sure, your new monthly payment will be all cute and adorable at first. It might even have your eyes and her smile. But faster than your fingers can mash the buttons on the calculator, your little payment will start to grow. It will blossom into orthodontist bills, insurance payments, plastic surgeon bills, and eventually into a fully grown second mortgage that hates you and refuses to live by your rules. The Dudes say that it's best to prepare yourself for that early. Otherwise you'll later be forced to destroy your liver with alcohol just to cope with the pressure. Luckily, as Science has shown us, the liver, like the appendix, serves no significant anatomical function.

It's Taxing

It's important to note that, like those phony charitable contributions on your income tax forms, children too are tax deductible. Your bundle of joy will be worth one tax exemption and subsequently qualifies you for a child tax credit. This can certainly help the cause during tax time, so don't forget to update your information as soon as your baby is born. (Don't mess with the IRS by doing it before the baby's born, though; they will find out and destroy you.)

Ironically, you can't put a price on love, but it's amazing how much that love will end up costing you. Much like your taxes, monthly baby payments might seem completely random, but they never actually go down. It's best to get used to that idea as soon as possible.

Midwifery and Other Politically Fashionable Births

Alternative births have received quite a bit of attention in recent years. Some people put a great deal of effort into keeping contemporary medicine at arm's length when delivering their baby. Alternative birthing, usually with a midwife, involves casting aside the notion that a sterile environment full of cold, unfeeling doctors and nurses is somehow beneficial. These pioneers of child birthing often look upon the modern medical establishment with distrust and contempt. They convince the women in their care of the same thing. Doctors just don't get it, and male doctors are often particularly frowned upon.

If your wife so chooses to disconsider germ-free environments and takes exception to the decades of training and medical experience of her doctor, then your local pseudo-physician midwife may be the way to go. You'll want to find one early in your pregnancy so she can start with the propagand...uh...er, we mean...guiding you down the path to enlightenment.

Alternative birthing covers just about every position and physical environment you can think of for having a baby. Modern painkillers and hospital procedures are the last resort. Some women might try to stand and squat to have the baby. Some might do it on their hands and knees. Some might even use one of those giant exercise balls. Midwives will do their best to accommodate whatever insane notion your wife might have about giving birth, as their main stated mission is to make birthing as comfortable and "natural" for your wife as possible. Interestingly, this is achieved by causing your wife as much pain as possible during delivery.

Some women might even be convinced to try to have the baby in a bathtub or some expensive, specially designed birthing version of a bathtub. This method of birthing is called the water birth or, as The Dudes call it, a birth in a vat of your own uterine goo and chunks. The theory is that it makes it less stressful and painful for the mother. The water somehow magically takes away a tiny portion of her pain and suffering. It's said that it's also less traumatic for the child to exit into a watery world similar to the womb.

Forgive us, but The Dudes, by nature, have a difficult time buying into this sort of new-age approach. If some-one could please point out which members of society were water-birthed, we'd be much obliged to see how fucking awesome they turned out to be. The Dudes think that being squeezed out of a hole that's the size of, well, an 8-pound baby's compressed skull, is going to be mind-wrenchingly traumatic no matter what the consistency of the outside world. Seriously, the baby's skull is actually made up of tiny bone pieces that overlap just so it can be compressed as much as possible to make it through the tiny exit. How's that for a beautiful miracle?

In light of that, you might think a Caesarian (C-section) birth would be better for the baby, as it avoids all the baby brain–squishing and wife pelvic expansion. It seems easy enough, right? The doctor "simply" cuts a gaping hole in your wife's abdomen and forcibly extracts the baby by hand. He then passes the baby to a nurse, who hands it off to your wife as a distraction while he attempts to close up the baby-sized hole he's just created.

Well, if you thought that, you'd be wrong. As it turns out, all that natural-birth compression on the baby's body actually forces various fluids out and kick-starts other important internal goings-on in the baby. You can talk to Science if you want the specifics. It can be noted here as well that the ultimate goal of midwives is actually to prevent the Caesarian at all costs: they see a Caesarian as a defeat. The Dudes reluctantly acknowledge that we agree with midwives about avoiding C-sections, but for an entirely different reason. C-sections tend to leave behind a giant scar. We know we're assholes, but sometimes it pays to be forward-thinking. However, if you're in this situation, you'll look like much less of an asshole if you just agree with the midwife and don't mention why you're agreeing with her.

If your wife craves the kind of personal attention that her family and doctors can't really give her, then a midwife might be just what the doctor ordered, even though a doctor never would. It seems conceivable that a midwife would form a greater bond with your wife than would her regular doctor. We've heard that women usually feel more comfortable discussing the more embarrassing details of pregnancy with them. You can see how this could be a wonderful time-saving benefit to *you* as well. She'll complain to the midwife about how the doctor never really seems to listen to her concerns during her (expensive) visits, and you won't have to be bothered with any of it. The midwife will in turn explain to your wife all about the evils of modern medicine and about how women have been having babies "naturally" in caves and covered wagons for hundreds of years.

The proponents of alternative birthing will tell your wife that hospitals are only there to make money, not to create a loving bond between mother, doctor, and child. They will expound on how pregnancy and birthing is a uniquely feminine and beautiful experience that should be enjoyed without the modern "comforts" provided by hospitals. Painkillers be damned for these modern-day heroes of pregnancy. However, please keep the ambulance engine warmed up, just in case.

The Dudes, however, are happy to keep at least one foot *outside* the cave at all times. We tend to err on the side of conventional Western medicine. So the baby gets a little morphine in the bloodstream before being born. Big deal. That just makes for a happier baby, in our opinion. It's true that painkilling drugs weren't around when our cave-dwelling ancestors were battling dinosaurs for supremacy, but neither was indoor plumbing. We sincerely doubt that pregnant, dinosaur-fighting cavewomen would have turned down either if they'd been available. The great thing about birthing alternatives, though, is that, like vegetarianism, they allow you to look condescendingly upon those who choose to eat delicious bacon—the bacon, in this case, being your wife's epidural.

So sit back and try to imagine your wife delivering your child in the comfort of your own bed. If you can picture that, then also picture a brand-new set of sheets and possibly a new mattress. Hiring a doctor-distrusting midwife for a home birth in your own bathtub may be the cost-cutting move you've been looking for, though. Yeah, sure, women used to have babies in caves and elevators and covered wagons, but if the term "infant mortality rate" means anything to you, you'll listen when The Dudes politely suggest you put on your Birkenstocks and hemp sweater, get in your Volvo, and drive your hippie ass to the hospital.

Ask The Dudes

Ask the Dudes

From: "sNuGg1z69"
To: "The Dudes" Dudes@DudesGuide.com
Sent: September 20

D3ar D00d5,
I mEt my wiFe in a cHat r0oM a few yEerz ago. Now shEez pRgninT aNd doEsN't hav n-e intrest in ChAtTiNg anym0r3. Pleez giVe m3 sum of ur great aDviCe. ?8°

Signed,
sNuGg1z69

Dear Internet Pervert,

Thanks so much for the great e-mail. We've been passing this one around quite a bit. And after weeks of thinking it over, we can honestly say, "What the fuck are you talking about?"

If we read this right, you met your wife online a few years ago. Well, whatever it is you're asking about, we think you should just feel lucky. Nowadays, a network news team would be waiting for you to show up to meet her and have the cops haul you off to jail on national television.

Sincerely,

The Dudes

📖 Myth vs. Fact 📖

Myth: You can tell a woman is pregnant merely from her maternal "glow."

Fact: You can tell a woman is pregnant from her ample behind, burrito in each hand, and the "I'm going to piss my pants" look on her face.

Myth: Fluctuating hormone levels can cause digestion problems during pregnancy.

Fact: Your wife's methane gas production could power Las Vegas for a week straight.

Myth: Exercise during pregnancy is highly recommended.

Fact: Exercise during pregnancy is usually avoided.

CHAPTER THREE

Weeks 10–13

Like your mom at the all-you-can-eat buffet, pregnancy keeps coming back for more. The wonders described in chapters 1 and 2 replay themselves for the next three to four weeks. And just when you think you can't take it anymore, it turns out you're right. You can't. To distract you from the inevitable, The Dudes have cooked up a little activity to help perk you up during the final stretch of the first trimester.

Dad-Libs

- Circle one word from each of the following numbered groups. For the advanced dude, be creative, and come up with your own disgusting nouns, verbs, etc.
- Read the story on page 67 aloud, plugging in the numbered words that you circled as you go along.
- Snicker like you're twelve again.

(1) Noun:
butt plug, jackhammer, crapper, fist, gerbil, porcupine, hooker, plunger, hot chick, midget, hot midget

(2) Food:
pizza, breakfast burrito, chicken wing, ketchup packet, live cockroach, Fruit Roll-Up, poo sandwich

(3) Exclamation:
Holy hell! Jesus H. Christ! WTF! Yeehaw! Hold my beer! Dee-am! No you dih-int! For fuck's sake!

(4) Form of Transportation:
magic carpet, Segway, fart-mobile, surfboard, wheelbarrow, three-legged mule, crotch rocket, monorail

(5) Magazine:
Penthouse, Boy's Life, High Society, MILF's Digest, Fat Chicks in Action, Cat Fancy

(6) Body Part:
left ball, neck meat, hemorrhoid, taint, extra toe, spleen, back fat, third nipple, conjoined twin

(7) Mechanical Object:
grain combine, fax machine, bowling ball return, ice-cream maker, particle accelerator, sewing machine

(8) Verb:
stroke, milk, pork, hump, mount, squeeze, moisten, grope, finger, soak

(9) Period of Time:
eons, one second, a trimester, for-fucking-ever, one rotation of the Earth, a New York minute

(10) Noun:
palmer, nutsack, puke pile, man hand, stupid head, testicle, rim job, jackass, beaver

(11) Noun:
camel toe, beotch, areola, ham, freedom fighter, douche bag, muff diver

(12) Fluid:
urine, synthetic motor oil, apple juice, pudding, saliva, beef drippings, biodiesel, butt juice

(13) Adjective:
smelly, salty, humid, crusty, vile, prehistoric, unorthodox, malformed, insulting, crude, dripping, slimy

(14) Orifice:
navel, gaper, sphincter, piehole, bunghole, cakehole, birthhole

(15) Adjective:
juicy, sexy, mucus-filled, hard-core, awesome, filthy, retarded, uncomfortable, dirty, thrill-a-minute

One day I was sitting on the (1) eating a (2). My wife interrupted me and asked if I'd like to go to her monthly prenatal appointment with her. "(3)" I shouted and quickly got up, spilling my (2) all over me. We hopped in our (4) and sped off to the doctor's office.

At the office, I read an old (5) to pass the time. There was a great article about how to avoid getting your (6) caught in a (7). Since I'd never gotten my (6) caught in a (7), I thought the info would come in handy someday. The nurse poked her head into the waiting room and said, "The doctor will (8) you now."

We waited in the examination room for what seemed like (9). The doctor came in and introduced himself. "Hi, I'm Dr. Harry (10)," he said. "You must be the husband of this beautiful young (11)." He promptly put some (12) on his hands for lubrication and inserted them into my wife's (13) (14).

"Everything seems to be progressing nicely," said Dr. (10). I'll see you back here next month for another (15) checkup.

CHAPTER FOUR

Weeks 14–17

Congratulations! You've made it through the first trimester. Just as you're getting used to this whole pregnancy thing, the fourth month bestows its gifts of weight gain, paranoia, and an unpredictable libido. The Dudes remind you to beware. There's a chance your wife will have similar, if not the exact same, symptoms.

News Womb

So you've successfully impregnated your wife (and probably on purpose). The Dudes offer heartfelt congratulations and possibly a high five. Your baby's mamma has managed to make it past the magical three-month marker mostly without incident, and it's highly likely that the pregnancy will "stick." If you weren't on Pregnancy Watch, then your pregnancy will probably still be a secret—a secret that you'll now need to share with the world.

Beginning on the ninety-first day, the elaborate process of spreading the news begins. For reasons unknown, never once in the history of the world has a woman simply said, "Mom and Dad, I'm pregnant." So, once your wife has officially given clearance to reveal the secret, you will have to come up with the requisite incredibly clever way to tell her parents the news. You will also undoubtedly decide that your kick-ass original news-spreading idea will be a puzzlelike gift that you will give to her parents. This will provide a slow and awkward-for-everybody way for them to attempt to figure out that she's pregnant. If this sounds confusing, that's because it is (we'll explain below). Furthermore, this will likely be done at a fancy restaurant that you never take them to, but her clueless folks will be unable to connect the huge, obvious dots.

[**NOTE:** Yes, we said *her* parents. In 98 percent of the cases we've observed, this is always the correct choice when it comes to whose parents to tell first. Her parents are first, no matter what, from now on. Remember that. Learn it. Live with it. Because if you don't, you're setting yourself up for a hell the likes of which you've never even dreamed of.]

If you're lucky, you can get away with a sonogram printout in a "Congratulations" card. This is the simplest way to go and should ensure that her parents take only fifteen to thirty minutes to figure out what it means. Even though an ultrasound printout is not an obscure medical document—a sort of reverse Rorschach inkblot on an oversized grocery receipt—being able to divine the image of an embryo about the size and relative shape of a peanut would be quite a feat even for the nonsenile of our population. Nonetheless, the mostly recognizable, fuzzy black-and-white image tends to scream, "You're looking at a fucking sonogram!" And unless you have a habit of taking your wife's parents out to dinner to show them your kidney stones, the signals are there.

Aside from the sonogram method, more elaborate methods of informing the in-laws include the gift of baby shoes, a baby doll, or an "I love my grandparents" bib. Bill recommended a tiny shirt embroidered with "You are probably too old and senile to figure out that this means your daughter is going to have a baby, thus making you the maternal grandparents." But his wife's lack of appreciation for awesome sarcasm, combined with the high per-word price for embroidery, steered him down the baby shoes route.

Up to an hour later and after you and your wife practically spell it out for them, it will dawn on them that she's pregnant. Then there will likely be laughing and crying and everything in between for the next half hour. You will get some awkward congratulations but will quickly be shoved to the back of the crowd so praise can be showered upon the real hero.

You and your wife will receive a barrage of questions. How far along is she? How long have you known? What's the due date? etc. You might be lucky enough to quietly slink out of the room to grab a beer while your wife fields all of these questions. The Dudes suggest that you try.

Father in Awe

It is at this point that it all starts falling apart for you. The Dudes like to call what's about to happen to you The Great Realization. Things are about to get painfully awkward, and if you're thinking that all of pregnancy is pretty much painfully awkward, you're right, but this is a special kind of awkward specifically reserved just for you. Unfortunately, there's not a damn thing you can do about it, either. Don't know what we're talking about? Well, here's how it played out for Scott.

Scott was at his in-laws' house when the clever card with the ultrasound photo was opened. Most of his wife's immediate family was on hand for the event. Once they finally realized what the card was telling them, twenty-seven minutes and thirteen seconds later, they began to congratulate Scott and his wife and comment on how original and clever the card was. As all the hugging and congratulating was tapering off, Scott's wife, her sisters, and her mother all went into another room to discuss the baby-related details. Thus, Scott was left alone with his father-in-law.[1]

Scott had always had a good relationship with his father-in-law, but now that they were alone, things didn't feel quite right. The conversation was short and awkward, and several times Scott thought he saw his father-in-law subtly shaking his head disapprovingly. The tension seemed to grow, and Scott was beginning to freak out a little. What about the good news? The upcoming grandchild? What about the clever card? Man, that card idea was awesome. Maybe his father-in-law thought Scott ripped off the card idea from that television show last week (he did). Shit. Maybe he knew? Maybe they all knew? They were in the kitchen, and the awkwardness and tension was causing Scott to panic. He offered to make his father-in-law a sandwich, thinking that might help get things back to normal. His father-in-law reluctantly accepted the offer. Scott proceeded to fashion a respectable sandwich. As he squirted some mayo onto the bread from the squeezable container, it finally hit Scott what was wrong, why his father-in-law had barely spoken a word to him since the card was opened.

---

1. Caution: If your wife has an older childless sister, that sister will probably fake excitement and then run to another room, sobbing uncontrollably, because her little sister got knocked up before her and stole all the pregnancy glory. Your wife and mother-in-law will be forced to console her for the next hour, thus allowing her to steal back the glory.

He realized that although his father-in-law was proud, Scott had just handed him undeniable proof that he had been having sweaty, perverted sex with his little girl.

Scott began to panic and fumble around the kitchen. In his panic, he began to blurt out things about mayonnaise and buns and proper meat placement, and the situation quickly deteriorated into a painfully awkward silence followed by an even more painfully awkward discussion about last week's Bears game. Scott was finally unintentionally rescued from the situation when his wife came in and demanded that he go to the store immediately and get her some chocolate-covered *anything* and a bag of Cheetos while she simultaneously devoured the symbolic sandwich Scott had made for her father.

To avoid the uncomfortable awkwardness resulting from The Great Realization, The Dudes suggest that after you've done your clever bit and they've heard the news, you leave your father-in-law alone for at least thirty minutes. Let the news sink in. He'll eventually get past it, but it's best if you're not trying to make him a sandwich at the time.

✓   **The Great Realization Quick Tip**   ✓

If you invite her parents out to dinner to break the news, The Great Realization will often be reduced to an uncomfortable glare from across the table.

Parental Notification

The Dudes have gone through the most painful aspects of pregnancy and lived to tell the story. While that might sound a tiny bit melodramatic, it doesn't make it any less true. Because we're your friends, we want to give you the valuable knowledge we've so painfully acquired so that you have a chance at avoiding as much of the pain as possible. And this would apply to how you spread the news beyond the in-laws.

So, the three-month wait is finally over, and you've told her parents. You might think that after that, the rest is going to be a cakewalk—just a few phone calls and everyone feels the love, right? WRONG! Like everything else in pregnancy, spreading the news should never be taken lightly or treated casually.

First of all, it's very important that you do this news spreading in the proper order. If you don't, you'll be forced to hear about it for years to come. This usually takes the form of sarcastic remarks from her grandmother, sisters, aunts, and friends during family get-togethers. Unless you live on different coasts, these get-togethers will probably happen with regular frequency. Our friend Ryan learned this lesson the hard way. On the day Ryan's wife gave the okay to tell everyone the wonderful news, he simply grabbed her address book, turned to the first page, and started calling people in alphabetical order.

People were happy to hear the news, of course, but they also had more questions. From several members of both of their families, he got the same unfortunate question: "Who else have you told?" Being the fool that he was, Ryan said, "I'm going alphabetically." That sealed his fate, because invariably the next question was, "Why did so-and-so find out before me?" Which was then followed by crying, followed by him saying, "But I was just going alphabetically, I didn't mean to...yeah, but..." We're sure you've got a good mental image of the hell he had to endure (and is still enduring). The best approach for spreading the news is one that The Dudes have dubbed The Wedding Table Approach (this can also apply to those of you outside the confines of wedlock; you'll just have to do more work).

Think back to your wedding. Do you remember having to go through the ordeal of ranking all of your friends and family by seating arrangement? The importance of the relative or friend was directly related to his or her physical distance from the bride and groom at the reception dinner. Remember the meticulously planned chart that looked similar to this?

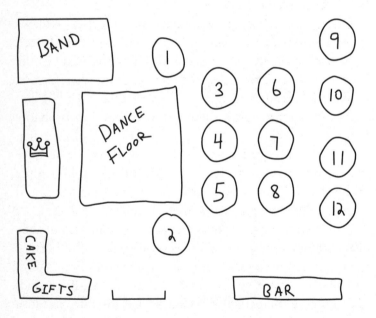

1. Bride's parents/siblings
2. Groom's parents/siblings
3. Bride's friends and their family members (I)

4. Bride's friends and their family members (II)
5. Bride's friends and their family members (Overflow)
6. Bride's coworkers
7. Bride's friends from grade school whom she doesn't talk to anymore
8. Friends of the bride's parents whom she knows
9. Friends of the bride's parents whom she doesn't know
10. Misc. unattractive relatives from out of state
11. Groom's *approved* friends and family members (please limit to four, plus their dates)
12. People who are only attending for the free booze

See, the closer they are, the more important they are. If your wife has saved any of the seating charts and other memorabilia from your wedding, get it out and look it over. That's very close to the exact order in which you should be telling people the good news. Her sister first, creepy Uncle Mark and his third soon-to-be-ex–old lady last. If you go with The Wedding Table Approach, years of annoying comments, in-law sarcasm, and irritation can be avoided. Down the road, you'll thank us. We even suggest you keep a copy of your wedding table diagram with you at all times. Who knows? It may come in handy again someday.

✓ **Notification Quick Tip** ✓

With subsequent pregnancies, other friends and family members will likely be informed *before* you.

Dude-on-Dude Hugging

Many of the circumstances surrounding pregnancy are very joyous. From the initial "we're pregnant" announcement to the hordes of relatives attacking your home, bringing gifts, love, and germs, pregnancy is filled with embraces both literal and figurative. Chances are you'll be faced with the uncomfortable circumstance of male-on-male contact. Worry not, however. The Dudes have a proven technique that will spare you the repeated anguish of this awkward situation. The following is the official Dudes-approved method for dude-on-dude hugging.

1. Firmly shake hands [Figure IIIa].
2. Position free left arm over opposing dude's right shoulder, with left hand on opposing dude's upper back. Opposing dude will follow suit [Figure IIIb].
3. Give two to four firm, open-handed pats on opposing dude's back.
4. Quickly release.

Alternate "Ethnic" Version: At Step 1, substitute "arm-wrestling style" underhand handshake [Figure IIIc]. At Step 3, substitute closed fist, patting with thumb side of fist, for open hand [Figure IIId].

We suggest you take a few hours to memorize the above technique, even practicing on a mannequin, CPR training dummy, etc., until you get it down pat. In the forthcoming months, you can relax, knowing how to properly address awkward same-sex contact.

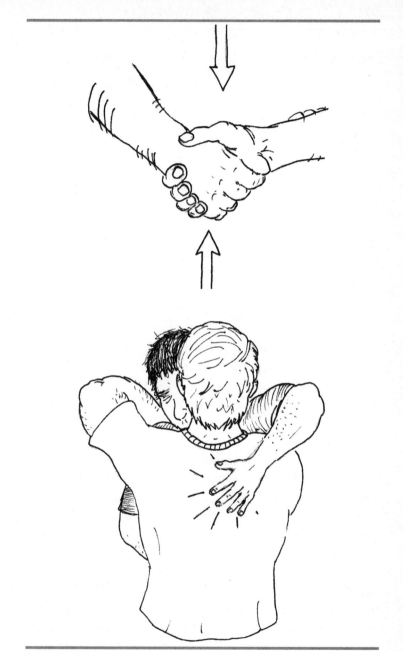

Figure III a (top), b (bottom)

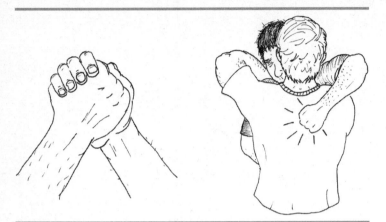

Figure III c (left), d(right), continued

Extrasexual Perception

As soon as the women in your wife's life learn that she's pregnant, they all become instant experts in the pseudoscience that is predicting your baby's gender. While our friend Science strongly frowns upon this ridiculous crap, he rarely says anything, because he's too busy trying to score with your wife's friends.

So while your wife's friends have Science distracted with their boobs, they'll convince your wife that they can actually predict with great accuracy the gender of the baby growing inside her. They'll further elaborate on how their foolproof prediction methods worked for their sisters, and cousins, and friends, and friends of friends.

The Dudes are here to help shed some light on the murky pregnancy gender-predicting pseudoscience underworld. We're here to expose the seedy underbelly of the actual pregnancy belly. We'll give you all the tools you need to debunk her bunk. In the end, though, we do recommend just letting her believe the nonsense. It's usually better that way.

There are five main stupid gender-prediction tests. Depending on the insanity of her friends and/or sisters, she'll be required to participate in at least three of them.

Morning Sickness

It is said that your baby's gender can be determined by the severity of your wife's morning sickness. If your wife has been puking uncontrollably for hours at a time, then supposedly she's going to have a girl. If her hurling was mild, it's a boy. Your wife will be able to find plenty of friends and family to swear that this is true.

Baby's Heart Rate

During your wife's prenatal OB/GYN visits, the doctor will often strap a microphone to her belly. He'll crank up the volume on the attached speaker, and your wife (and possibly you) will be able to hear the baby's heartbeat. You'll be in awe at the miracle of life that she's carrying around inside her. What you might not realize, though, is that your baby is actually trying to tell you its gender.

If the heartbeat is fast, then your baby wants you to know that it's a boy. If the heartbeat is slow, then your baby wants you to start saving for her wedding. From what we understand, 140 beats and above per minute is considered boy territory. Unfortunately, the guiding hand of Science is still trying to grab your wife's friend's juggs, so he'll be of little use. Thus, the heart-rate theory will be interpreted as fact.

Chinese Fertility Chart

As you might have guessed, The Dudes tend to put a great deal of their faith in the wonders of Eastern medicine. We believe that shark-penis burritos will increase the size of your hang-down by at least 50 percent. This goes double for panda bear testicles and anything having to do with a tiger. It follows logically, then, that we would put much stock in the Chinese fertility chart, which is incredibly popular among expectant mothers. Cross-referencing the month of conception with the age of the mother will yield the new baby's gender. Your wife's friends will claim that the chart worked on her friend's friend last year, so it must be accurate. The Dudes would comment further on this, but we haven't finished our burrito yet.

Pencil Test

The pencil test is basically the Ouija board of pregnancy. Your wife is instructed to tie a string to the eraser end of a pencil. She is then supposed to dangle the pencil over her belly while keeping her hand perfectly still. The pencil tip moving in a strong circular motion is a clear indication that the benevolent pregnancy spirits on the other side think she'll have a girl. Alternatively, if the pencil swings back and forth, the spirits think it's a boy.

Like the Chinese fertility chart, your wife's friend will assure her that this test also worked for a friend of a friend.

Drano Test

Yes, you read that correctly. The *Drano* Test. This test will have your wife living out her dream of becoming a world-renowned chemist, all at the possible expense of your baby's DNA as she breathes in the caustic fumes of urine mixed with crystal Drano. We can't even believe that we're writing this, but we'd hate for you to be misled, so here's how one version of this insanity works:

Materials List:
1 glass jar
2 tablespoons crystal Drano
2–3 ounces of her urine, preferably her first of the day
1 dose of complete insanity

First, your wife will take the 1 dose of complete insanity. She will then add two tablespoons of crystal Drano to the empty glass jar. Then, if all went well, she will pour the 2 to 3 ounces of morning pee into the glass jar and run like hell so as not to inhale the noxious fumes.

After the chemicals react, she will observe the color. If the mixture has turned brownish, then it's a guaranteed boy. If there has been no color change, then the magic potion will have predicted a girl. We're guessing that the Drano Test has something to do with hormones and chemicals and shit, but with all these fumes, we're having a hard time concentrating. Aside from now knowing the gender of your baby, your wife can then pour the whole horrible mixture down the drain and clean it out.

Rotating Metal Disk Test

Not to be overshadowed by a strong tradition of stupidity, The Dudes have come up with our own test. All you'll need is a small, circular metal disk and a pinch of gumption for this one. Mark the disk on one side (a coin works well due to its distinctive markings) and place it on the fingernail side of the pregnant woman's thumb. Have her quickly move her thumb upward, or "flip" the "coin," causing it to rotate in the air. If the metal disk lands on the marked (heads) side, it's a boy. If it lands on the unmarked (tails) side, think pink!—you'll be having a girl. Or vice versa!

The Dudes can say with sarcastic confidence that the test we made up works just as well as the other ones involving string, Asian superstitions, or harmful chemicals. We can also say that if your wife has patience enough to wait until her next ultrasound, the technician can just look for a penis.

Sexual Tension

Pretty much every dude has a preference for the baby's gender, and you will inevitably be asked what your preference is. It's perfectly acceptable to want a girl more than a boy, or vice versa. This is obviously not an indication of how much you will love the baby or an indication that you will abandon your baby in disgust if *he* turns out to be a girl.

You know this. The Dudes know this. Unfortunately, other key people don't seem to get it. Sometimes they even seem a bit offended if you choose one gender over the other. Take Scott's mother-in-law. She would always ask him what he wanted, just in case he had changed his mind since the last time she asked. The conversation would go like this 100-fucking-percent of the time:

Mother-in-law: "So, what are you hoping for?"
Scott: "I'm hoping for a boy."
Mother-in-law: "Oh, well, that's nice."

Scott: (awkward silence)
Mother-in-law: "Well, as long as it's healthy."

As long as it's healthy...Please allow The Dudes to translate that for you:

"How dare you be selfish enough to disregard the health of the baby by being so selfishly concerned about what gender *you* selfishly want."

Now there's a revelation *and* an insult all packed into one overly concerned–sounding line. Not only does it suggest that Scott's desire for a boy automatically means he doesn't give a shit if it's an unhealthy girl, but it completely invalidates the original question because it seemingly has no correct answer at all. You will hear this "as long as it's healthy" line over and over again from various people until you actually do find out the gender via ultrasound or actual birth. The Dudes suggest that you bury your frustration deep down inside and finish off the conversation with, "of course, as long as it's healthy."

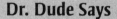

Dr. Dude Says

"The odds of having twins are about 3 in 100.
Interestingly, so is the failure rate of the birth control
pill. This makes the odds of accidentally having
twins 9 in 1,000."

Mayday, I'm Going Down

The second-trimester months bring with them a new series of hurdles for you to contemplate jumping over. Sometimes you'll jump, and sometimes you'll puke in your own mouth a little bit and then still jump anyway.

After three long months of relentless nonsexual activity, something truly amazing happens. The first trimester usually goes out with a "bang." Luckily for you, you've reached that pregnancy twilight where there's a slight chance of some seriously sweet sex. The Dudes refer to this as your Sexual Oasis of Sex, or SOS.

During this SOS, she's just barely showing, her hormones have leveled off to the point where she's not constantly puking, and she might even have extremely sensitive erogenous zones (read: crotch). We theorize that this is Nature's way of rewarding you for your patience during the first trimester's masturbation marathon. (It also is probably the period that gave all the authors of those lame pregnancy books your wife read the idea that pregnancy is a sensual, nine-month lovefest.) But just as soon as your SOS appears, it is gone.

Bill had taken the first three-month dry spell as a hint that he was facing more like a nine-month sexual drought. He failed to pick up on the hints that his wife was dropping that she was, sexually speaking, her old self again, and he missed his window of opportunity. The Dudes urge you to take advantage of an SOS, because this will be the last time for several months that you'll be able to get any without the aid of some sort of hoisting apparatus. Don't miss this once-in-a-pregnancy chance or, like Bill, you could be left standing in the rain on the side of the road, holding your boner and crying.

One of the advantages of an SOS is how carefree it is. As far as we know, unless you're Irish, you can't possibly impregnate her again while she's pregnant. So it's the first time in your life so far that you're guaranteed sex without consequences. (In the coming months, though, consequences quickly turn to discharge, so strike while you can.) As awesome as that freedom sounds, it does come at a price. Pregnancy has its own special way of making awesome stuff much less awesome. It's sometimes hard to enjoy not worrying about knocking your wife up when you suddenly find yourself thinking about how uncomfortably close your porn-star unit is to your unborn child's face. That's some serious psychological trauma that'll guarantee years of therapy down the road. Think of the *children*! (Just not during sex).

Your wife's belly is just starting to grow, but her tits have gotten a big head start. You remember from chapter 1 that your wife began to sprout Pamela Anderson boobs and that, like Pam's, you aren't allowed to touch them? Like all things pregnancy, what seemed like a nice little bonus is about to turn ugly. Unable to support their growing mass, her boobs are going to start heading southward. She's just a few months or years away from a pair of "National Geographic specials" (and the boob is taking the nipple down with it): hearken back to the nipple chart from chapter 1, which clearly shows that, as her juggs grow, so do her nipples. Now it's time for her nipples to start changing color. They become dark, angry, and foreign and tend to get in the way of that whole visual stimulation thing that you were counting on so much.

The Dudes have read most of the sex chapters of the pregnancy books that our wives got. Yeah, we could have read other chapters too, but that's pretty much all we were interested in. We've reached the conclusion that the sex chapters in those pregnancy books for women are mostly full of lies and half-truths. They are misleading at best. Furthermore, those chapters are specifically designed to fool the husband into thinking that everything's going to be just fine. Well, we're here to tell you that it's not going to be fine. It's going to be the opposite of fine. It's going to be *not* fine.

From here on out, it's an uncomfortable downhill ride on the pregnancy sex train. It gets even worse because as she's expanding, your hope of any normal version of sex is doing the total opposite of expanding. It's *not* expanding. When our wives were pregnant, we could see where things were going. We could see the inevitable impossibility of normal, nonawkward intercourse, and it choked us up a little. Seriously, don't ever think for a second that you can beat pregnancy. It's had millions of years to figure out how to screw you. You've only had a few months. You're no match for it.

Upset Stomach

Late in the fourth month, your wife will start to notice her budding belly expansion. She'll think it's cute and stand in front of the mirror for minutes (or hours) at a time, looking at it from all different angles. She'll poke and prod it, wondering what it's going to look like in five months. She'll be slightly bummed that her pants don't quite fit anymore. Conversely, she may be oddly bummed out if she's *not* showing yet. Our friend Brandon experienced this strange, Catch-22–like situation himself. His wife was not looking forward to an expanding waistline but was frustrated because she didn't look pregnant. It just hurts our brains thinking about it. In order to stave off subsequent brain cramps, Brandon came up with a great line that deployed her own pregnancy powers against her like a kind of gestational judo. It's a brilliant line that The Dudes are happy to pass along to you.

> *Wife:* [tearing up] "I'm so upset; my favorite jeans don't fit anymore. I have to use a rubber band to keep them closed."
>
> *Brandon:* [dripping with sarcasm] "Hrmmmm. Let's see here. I'm pretty sure there's a small human life growing inside of you right now. Yeah, weird."
>
> *Wife:* "You're the greatest husband ever. How about I make out with my girlfriends for you?"
>
> *Brandon:* [wry, satisfied smile]

Works like a charm every single time. We can learn a lot from Brandon and his masterful application of sarcasm. Or we can fill our spank banks with images of Brandon's wife making out with her hot friends. Either way, problem solved every single time.

Nonetheless, since medical professionals frown upon the notion of utilizing a corset during pregnancy, The Dudes urge you to accept the inevitable. What starts as a quaint little bump will continue to grow exponentially from here on out. While she's poking at it, trying to see if she can feel the baby, you need to be aware that this is the last time you're ever going to see her body the way it is now. The Dudes don't mean to be dramatic, but we can't stress this enough. We also sincerely hope you took our advice and took pictures, like Brandon did, when you had the chance. (You're now aware of the concept of belly expansion. But were you aware of the phenomenon of ass expansion? Your wife's ass grows in direct proportion to her belly.)

| 🚐 | **Dr. Dude Says** | 🚐 |

"An occasional glass of wine during pregnancy won't do any harm to the fetus. It may even have the added bonus of making your wife think you're attractive."[1]

Change of a Dress

The cute novelty of your wife's expanding belly will quickly turn to panic as she becomes unable to fit into her regular clothes. To help herself get over this, she'll talk to her friends and sisters about her options. They'll tell her to try to look on the bright side, which will happen to be that she gets to go shopping for new clothes. Shopping tends to have the magical effect of making your wife happy while making your bank account sad. And if your wife does not think sweatpants, sweatshirts, muumuus, togas, or any other clothing that can be made out of old bedsheets are acceptable ladies' fashion, then it's inevitable that your wallet is in for a workout. It's all for the greater good though, right? Right.

As you know, The Dudes are here to help you deal with her dealing with her pregnancy. The subject of maternity clothes probably doesn't seem like that big a deal compared to everything else. You're correct, but in the interest of full disclosure, there are a few points we'd like to make you aware of before you try to stumble your way through some potentially awkward situations.

The Dudes can say with great confidence that all maternity clothes look like crap. Their primary function is to do their

---

1. Note: Dr. Dude is not an actual doctor.

best at hiding her expansion. Their secondary function is to make her as comfortable as possible while still accomplishing their primary function. Making her as comfortable as possible usually involves some sort of giant, expandable, marsupiallike pouch for her belly to fit into. This is then followed by a layer or two of flowery material to cover up said pouch.

Although it didn't happen to us, we feel great sympathy for those of you who are about to be dragged to the maternity-clothes store in the mall to help her pick out some outfits. We know you'd rather be doing anything but that, but be strong. And feel free to tell her that she looks cute when she shows you some of her new maternity clothes. With the help of Science, we have determined that "You look cute" is the optimal response to her question about how she looks in maternity clothes. Do this as often as needed.

You might also notice the appearance of the "mystery bag" of maternity clothes around this time. In addition to shopping for new maternity clothes of her own, your wife will get the mystery bag. The bag is like the football of pregnancy. It gets passed around by your wife's friends and family, and each person who gets it contributes the maternity clothes she doesn't need anymore. Keep in mind that no matter how ridiculous some of the clothes in the bag might be, they will ultimately save you money. Again, "You look cute" comes in very handy here as well.

Making Weight

And now we'd like to address a point that is often overlooked by lesser pregnancy books and is of crucial importance to The Dudes. While your wife is eating for two for nine months, you will be too. Some refer to Dad's weight gain as "sympathy pounds." That's misleading. We think "trophy pounds" or "pride pounds" is a much more appropriate term. Hell, you've done your work; now it's time to reap the rewards by gorging yourself. Your wife can only look on lovingly as your steady weight gain helps to fulfill your evolutionary destiny of becoming a father and thus never being attractive to another woman again. Ever.

After the baby comes, your wife may try to lose weight and get back into shape. The Dudes suggest you keep those pounds. They're yours, man. You earned 'em. After all, you're no longer a man, you're a dad. Biceps make way for bald spots. Pecs are to be replaced by prostate problems. You're basically a couple stomachaches away from your first colonoscopy. It's time to stand proud and show the world your big, buttery smile, fatty.

Ask The Dudes

Dear Dudes,

I've noticed lately that my wife is preoccupied with her pregnancy and seems to be neglecting both my emotional and my physical needs. Is this normal? Is there anything I can do about it?

Sincerely,
Some Wuss

Dear SW,

Wow, where do we even start? We recommend taking a romantic shower with your wife. If you're lucky, you can get her to wash your huge vagina for you. Proper care of your huge vagina is a must during your wife's pregnancy. Remember, you've only got the one huge vagina, and if you take care of it, it'll take care of you. Hope that helps.

Sincerely,

The Dudes

Suburban Legends

The litany of hormones coursing through your wife's body starts to find its groove during month four. In addition to random episodes of crying, dizziness, and paranoia, your wife will start to experience more organized episodes of insanity, as her hormones start to team up to conspire against her and, thusly, you. The foremost of these episodes is The Car Seat Incident. You can tell it's officially party time at the asylum when she first experiences the thought of leaving the baby's car seat, with baby strapped in it, on the roof of the car, only to realize miles down the road what she's done. This gold standard of pregnancy paranoia will show up over and over for the next six months, invading her thoughts and dreams. This particular episode is so universal for pregnant women that in some cat-eating parts of the world, a woman isn't even considered officially pregnant until she experiences it.

While The Car Seat Incident seems to be common among pregnant women, many other ridiculous delusions and cautionary tales are handed down by crazy old aunts in creepy, witchy voices. Some examples:

■ *Curse caffeine!* Chain-smoking doctors of the 1950s and '60s believed that caffeine could cross the placenta and enter the baby's brain, causing it to explode. Interestingly, these were the same doctors who were prescribing thalidomide for morning sickness, with nonhilarious results. Nowadays doctors say caffeine is fine, but keep it to three or four cups of coffee per day.

■ *A smelly mom-to-be a healthy baby brings!* "No baths" is an old pregnancy rule that probably originated in eastern Europe, where bathing in general is frowned upon. Doctors now qualify this outdated advice by adding no *hot* baths. Even this is not so much for the baby's sake as it is for the fainting-prone mom. Nonetheless, "stanky" is not a word you want to add to the already long list of your wife's unfortunate pregnancy side-effects.

■ *Dye not your hair when with child!* This one actually had some validity to it...thirty years ago. From 1950 until 1975, most women got their hair dyed with gasoline- and plutonium-infused coloring agents, resulting in the current generation of Kenny Chesney fans (at least, that's the only way we can explain it). Hair-dyeing technology has since developed less-caustic chemicals to achieve that perfect hooker-with-a-heart-of-gold look that's so popular with today's modern woman, although some doctors still recommend letting her roots grow out during the first trimester.

■ *Hands up and the baby gets it!* Like the myth of Walt Disney's cryogenically frozen body or the myth of Barry Bonds *not* using steroids, this one's so bad it's good. The notion that somehow an expectant mother raising her hands above her head will cause the umbilical cord to wrap around the baby's neck is a classic. What's even crazier is that it's 100 percent true.

DICs of Hazzard

It was around month four that Sensitive Guy approached Scott and asked him if he'd heard of the video titled *Honey, I'm Pregnant Too!* Shuddering, Scott indicated that he hadn't and braced himself, because he knew Sensitive Guy was about to hand him the copy he'd been unsuccessfully trying to hide behind his back. Holding out the old, worn-out–looking VHS tape, Sensitive Guy told Scott about how this video had helped him and his wife become closer during their pregnancies. Scott reluctantly took it and tried to read the back cover, which Sensitive Guy had already started reciting verbatim.

Apparently the video was about the more sensitive side of pregnancy. It claimed to be "45 minutes of inspiration, information, and entertainment." Even better, it was hosted by television's John Schneider, aka Bo Duke from *The Dukes of Hazzard*. It was apparently made during a stretch of his career when it was hard for him to find work. Sensitive Guy said that it had a "tear jerker" of an ending when the main couple's baby was brought into the world as the cameras rolled. Sensitive Guy actually said to Scott, "The end really delivers," causing Scott to shudder and gag slightly.

Scott was skeptical—not just about that contents of the video but about actually having a working VCR somewhere in his house. He told Sensitive Guy that he'd "definitely think about watching it." Satisfied with that, Sensitive Guy went back to his desk.

Scott ended up giving the tape to Foreign Guy, even though Foreign Guy was single and had few girlfriend prospects. Nonetheless, he was overly appreciative, as Foreign Guy always seems to be. "Thank you so much for gift, Scott. *Dukes for Hazzard* is number-one show to viewing in my country." Scott didn't have the heart to tell him that it wasn't an episode of the Dukes but laughed to himself at the thought of a surprise appearance by a "Cooter" of sorts during the tear-jerking finale of the video.

📖 Myth vs. Fact 📖

Myth: Pregnancy is your father-in-law's definitive proof that you "deflowered" his little girl.
Fact: His little girl was "deflowered" by three to twenty-five guys before you ever even met her.

Myth: Maternity clothes are cute and practical.
Fact: Muumuus are comfy and affordable.

Myth: The Chinese fertility chart can point out your baby's gender.
Fact: The Chinese fertility chart can point out your gullibility. (Note: also works with fortune cookies.)

Myth: Spreading the news of pregnancy is a joyous occasion.
Fact: Spreading the news to the wrong people first will cause more marital and familial strife than can be reasonably imagined. Also, you're stupid.

Myth: Pregnant women want to have sex with you during the second trimester.

Fact: Pregnant women want to have sex with George Clooney throughout the second trimester.

Myth: Partners of pregnant women often add unwanted pounds during pregnancy.

Fact: Husbands of pregnant women lose their will to give a crap about a lot of stuff.

CHAPTER FIVE

Weeks 18–22

Congratulations! Through all the nagging, weight gain, paranoia, butt growth, and temper tantrums, you may have missed the fact that you've made it to the halfway point (you may also have missed your wife exhibiting similar pregnancy symptoms). In an effort to see where you stand physically and emotionally, Science has helped us put together the following questionnaire for you. Pick one word from each of the following groups of words that best describes how you're feeling. Don't worry—there are no right or wrong answers:

a) calm   a) excited   a) light-headed
b) uneasy   b) indifferent   b) dizzy
c) panicked   c) depressed   c) unconscious

a) confident   a) proud   a) halcyon
b) confused   b) unsure   b) palpitant
c) WTF?   c) Oh my God.   c) timorous
                            What have I
                            done?

a) masculine	a) regular	a) chartreuse
b) neuter	b) blocked up	b) magenta
c) totally gay	c) crapping my pants	c) aquamarine

Scoring:

Award yourself 1 point for each *a* answer, 2 points for each *b* answer, and 50 points for each *c*. Here's how your results break down:

10–20 points: not screwed
20–49 points: somewhat screwed
50+ points: totally and completely screwed

Analysis:

50 percent of all men who took this quiz scored at least 250 points.

The other 50 percent got a creepy *Cosmo* vibe and wisely skipped the quiz altogether.

Sexual Preference

For a statistical survey we did among three dudes we know, each of them admitted that they had a gender preference when it came to their unborn child. Although we've forgotten most of what they said, we do remember this: one said that he'd like a girl for the first fourteen or so years, then a boy for the rest. He said that girls were cute and fun until the teenage years, when you've got to start kicking the crap out of their loser boyfriends. As fun as that sounds, you have to remember that no matter what you do, she'll eventually marry one of those guys, and guess who's going to be paying for the wedding? He pointed out that a boy at that age is sort of on autopilot. As long as he stays out of jail, avoids the aforementioned beatings by his girlfriend's father, and becomes successful in all the ways you weren't, things will work out just fine. It's an interesting theory and one that we fully subscribe to.

Unfortunately, the above doesn't change (or have anything to do with) the fact that you will eventually be presented with the option of knowing if it's going to be a boy or a girl. Ultrasound is a wonderful thing, and its implications must be carefully considered. If you do find out, your wife could have as many as five months to shop for the unborn girl or boy. Conversely, if you don't find out, she might hold off buying anything until after the baby is born. By that time she might have a better idea of what she actually needs, instead of what she thinks Dude Jr. will like. Also, if you do decide to find out, a strange thing might begin to happen. You might start to personify your wife's stomach. Maybe you'll name it. Maybe you'll use a different voice around it. Maybe you'll even order separate meals for it. Maybe your wife will start saying, "Okay, I'll see you later, honey. [Your baby's name] and I will miss you" (and as creepy as that might sound now, it will seem perfectly normal to you when it happens, and you'll think nothing of it).

On the other hand, if you decide not to find out, there are other things you'll have to deal with. For one, you'll undoubtedly get a ton of mint green–colored baby gifts from your friends and family, gifts that will end up being useless because they—as your wife will be happy to tell you—"just don't fit in" with the rest of the baby gear. What that means to you is more shopping.

Another potential hazard of waiting to find out is that you'll have to deal with your wife's occasional frustrated outbursts. It's amazing how many color-based decisions she'll think she has to make, and make right friggin' now. Not knowing the sex of the baby can get in the way of many of these decisions. What outfit do you bring to the hospital? (Bring two, a pink and a blue.) What color should the baby's room be? (Just paint it yellow, for crap's sake.) It could be anything. Good luck.

No matter the sex, though, it's never too early to think about all of your shortcomings and the fact that this is your opportunity to totally make up for them. If you're going to have a boy, think about all the sports you sucked at, then imagine all the great sports awards he'll win to make you look good. You might even want to consider becoming his coach to further grease the gears of justice. He can look forward to cool sports like baseball, basketball, football, hockey, wrestling, lacrosse, etc. (and if it's a girl, softball).

Beyond sports, there are innumerable other shortcomings that your child can help you make up for. If it's a boy, he can

- become both a fighter pilot *and* a rock star.
- finish the 72-ounce sirloin "Steak-a-saurus" and win a free T-shirt and the admiration of all the townsfolk.
- cure the STD that you've been secretly carrying around.
- win a poker tournament.
- bang his hot high school history teacher.
- acquire actual knowledge.

If it's a girl, she can

- hook you up with a continual, free supply of Girl Scout cookies.
- um . . . other important girl stuff that we can't think of right now.

Nonetheless, your child will no doubt have a wealth of shortcomings, unfinished projects, and/or regrets to choose from.

Aural Exam

An important pregnancy milestone is the sonogram, or ultrasound, taken around week twenty. It's ordered by the doctor to check on the baby's progress and general health, but is also highly anticipated because the grainy image can reveal your baby's gender. As we mentioned, The Dudes find this most helpful. Knowing your baby's gender will make life easier for you in many ways—from choosing your baby's name to registering for baby shower gifts.

Couples sometimes opt to get in touch with their inner Amish and decide not to find out the sex of the baby. The expectant mother might say something like, "Hezekiah and I want to wait until birth to find out. It will give me more incentive to push the baby out." Well, we've got news for you, sister: without having ever experienced a single contraction in our lives, we can assure you that when the baby decides to come out, the thought of not wanting to push it out is hilariously inconceivable.

We've often heard the equally ridiculous explanation "We're waiting to find out because we want to be surprised."

Guess what? The result will be just as surprising at twenty weeks as it will be at forty weeks. It's not like you get another possible outcome—boy, girl, or leprechaun—if you wait.

Why not take this element of surprise a step further? Why not wait until your androgynous child's first birthday to take a look-see? After all, it will make looking forward to the birthday party that much more exciting for friends and family. Better yet, why not wait until he/she graduates from high school to find out? Wow, then you'll be really surprised, huh?!?

Feeling our sarcasm? Good.

The actual ultrasound will be performed by an ultrasound "technician," not to be confused with "actual medical professional." For all we know (and we know a lot), any knucklehead with a GED and $250 can get his ultrasound technician certification and a free T-shirt after completing a one-day online cyberclass. Of course, after sitting through a five-minute ultrasound ourselves, The Dudes are convinced we could do it pretty easily, and likely way better than the Ultrasound College of America T-shirt–clad, mouth-breathing technician.

So, based on our experiences, without further ado, here is the step-by-step Dudes' Guide to Sonic Imaging:

1. Procure sonogram machine.
2. Squirt blue ultrasound goo onto subject's belly.
3. After subject squirms from uncomfortably cold blue ultrasound goo, say, "Oh, I should have warned you it would be cold."
4. Move magic ultrasound thingy randomly about subject's goo-covered belly until you see grainy, babylike images on the sonogram display.

5. Take some measurements that nobody cares about because all that's wanted is a crotch shot.
6. Say, "Uh oh. The legs are closed. I guess baby doesn't want you to know yet if it's a boy or a girl. Good thing your husband took a day off work to be here for nothing."
7. Hastily wipe blue ultrasound goo off subject's belly, accidentally leaving some to soak through her shirt.
8. Bill insurance company $1,000.

Like a lot of parents-to-be find out, Bill's first fetus decided not to give up its genital secret at the ultrasound. Fortunately, the technician couldn't seem to find a fourth heart chamber, either. As heart chambers are very important for humans to be able to live, another ultrasound was scheduled for two weeks later to have another look at this potentially serious defect. Bill knew better, though; the kid was clearly screwing with them. He quietly celebrated to himself as the ol' three-chamber heart trick failed to keep him from eventually learning his daughter's gender two weeks later. (Note: it was a girl.)

Conversely, everybody knows a guy whose cousin had a friend whose boss got the wrong gender from the ultrasound. It happens. In fact, it happened to Scott's cousin's friend's boss. There's really no consolation or advice to offer in this situation, since you won't be finding out how screwed you are until four months down the road anyway. Just know that the pink princess sheets in your new baby boy's crib won't make him gay. It's an overbearing mother who does that.

Dr. Dude Says

"My old Phi Delta Epsilon fraternity brother just found out his wife is having triplets. That's what I'm talkin' about, Noonski! Phi Delts RULE!!"

Return to Gender

Many husbands of pregnant women are not able to attend the twenty-week ultrasound, when their unborn child's gender is magically revealed. They are at their jobs, working for a living, attempting to stave off the impending financial crisis. Fortunately, ultrasound technicians are aware of your commitment to work your fingers to the bone to build a happy home for your growing family. They have devised a technique to reveal the news to both you and your wife simultaneously after your hard day of backbreaking labor. It's called sex in an envelope.

Our civil rights–activist friend Antwon has been there. His wife accidentally scheduled her ultrasound on the day of a very important march to City Hall. That morning, as Antwon grabbed his megaphone to head off to work, she reminded him about the important appointment at Dr. Az-Hakeem's office that day. But like many hardworking dudes, Antwon had commitments to his coworkers and the community that had to be kept.

At the appointment later that day, Antwon's wife asked the ultrasound technician to write down the baby's still-secret gender and put it in an envelope so she and Antwon could learn the news together. Problem solved.

After a late-night press conference to announce brutality lawsuits against the city and its police department, Antwon returned home exhausted. He excitedly removed his bow tie, put on some smooth jazz, and opened the envelope with his wife, bringing an exciting end to an otherwise daunting day.

The Name Game

Naming your baby can be a fun and exciting experience. It can also be a nerve-wracking pain in the ass. As with most things that affect your ability to cope with reality, this, too, depends mostly on your wife.

Maybe you both were in perfect agreement and had your boy and/or girl names picked out even before conception. Maybe you're one of *those* couples. If you are, that's just great. We're all proud of you. Now put down the book, get in your stupid Volvo, and go buy another disgustingly cute outfit for little Alexis, because you have no business reading this book in the first place. However, if you aren't one of the above-mentioned couples, The Dudes have some potentially helpful advice for you. Advice that, if you're like us, you'll probably ignore, but advice nonetheless.

Now, it's of utmost importance to remember that your child's name is potentially one of the greatest gifts and/or curses that you can give as a parent. That's a responsibility that shouldn't be taken lightly. The first and most important thing to think about is high school. Kids are mean, and since there are a lot of kids in high school, it logically follows that it's a mean place. Given that, you need to think about all the potential nicknames that these brutal little bastards can come up with. You have to be smarter than them and scru-

tinize each potential name as though you w
student. Here is an example of what we're ta.

Recently, a friend of ours and his wife wei.
think of names for their baby. They had found out t..
ultrasound that it was going to be a boy. They thought long
and hard and finally, in a frenzied burst of creativity, they
decided on John. John sounds like a fine name—good,
solid, manly. Sure, high school kids could probably come
up with a few things, but nothing that really sticks.

They both liked the name John, so they set about deciding on a middle name. Since the hard part was over, our
friend Ron had pretty much let his wife handle the middle
name. Huge mistake. Huge. After some trial and error, his
wife decided that she absolutely loved the name Thomas
for a middle name. That's right—she wanted to name their
baby boy John Thomas.

Now, it is your duty as the father of your child to recognize the horror that would have unfolded if our friend had
allowed his wife to name their boy John Thomas. It is your
duty to intervene and put a stop to ugly situations like this
before they get out of hand. Because, as you well know,
"John Thomas" is a euphemism for penis.

Aside from what The Dudes call the High School Factor,
there is another thing you need to be aware of when picking
a name: current trends. You might feel the urge to be creative
with your child's name—you might want to be different for
the sake of being different. Well, all we can say is don't. That's
what every other asshole on the planet is thinking too.

Being different for the sake of being different will only
result in one of two things: either your kid will have some
stupid hippie crap name or your kid will have a common
name with a stupid spelling. I mean, think about all the

different freakin' ways you can spell Kaitlyn, Katelin, Kait-elin, Caitlynn....Both situations should be avoided at all costs. Bill went to one of those little-kid gym classes with his kid—the kind where all the little kids have name tags on their backs. There were three little boys there, all from different parents, and their names were as follows: Ayden, Brayden, and Jayden. People, please...seriously. Don't try to be cute or clever or original. It *will* backfire.

♀   The Name-Game Evaluation   ♀

The Dudes have come up with a simple test to help determine how stupid the name you've chosen actually is. Write the name your wife thinks is so awesome in the blank provided below, and follow the rules to see how wrong she probably is.

1. Does the name have an endless possibility of spellings (Briana, Breanna, Bree-Anna)? yes—50 pts, no—0 pts
2. Does the supposedly cool name end with an "en" sound (Fallon, Cameron, Landon, Carson, etc.)? yes—50 pts, no—0 pts
3. Is the name a somewhat common name that is purposely misspelled (Jennipher, Treesa, or Jaysen)? yes—25 pts for each different letter, no—0 pts
4. Does the name sound close to a normal name, but isn't (Aris, Kristeem, or Josten)? yes—50 pts, no 0—pts
5. Will your child be the only person in the world with this name? yes—100 pts, no—0 pts

Now add up your total. If your total is greater than 1, you are probably dangerously close to embarrassing yourself and your unborn child. The higher the total, the more embarrassment.

Bonus round: *If the name you've chosen for your daughter utilizes "ie" or "ee" instead of the standard "y" (ex. Sandie, Sindee, Aimee), she will likely eventually be featured on a* Girls Gone Wild Spring Break *DVD. And won't that make you proud?*

If there's one thing we've noticed about everyone, ever, it's that their baby name suggestions will be the exact same suggestions that you and your wife already made fun of and decided against. Not only that, but they will undoubtedly grimace at the name you've chosen while pretending that they like it. It would be best to avoid this by telling people that you haven't picked out a name yet and to never ask you again or you'll punch them in the neck.

Now, you might think that we're hypocrites for telling you to ignore other people's horrible name suggestions, then suggesting our own, but you'd be wrong. We're hypocrites for several entirely different reasons. Now go on and name your child with these things in mind. Remember, the name you give your child is something he or she will have to live with until he or she is legally old enough to go to court and have it changed to something that doesn't suck. Try to think of names that command authority and respect. The Dudes would like to suggest a few names to get you started.

Boy Names:

- Blake Armstrong
- Max Power

- Trent Steel
- Trevor Hightower

Girl Names:

- Cassandra Irons
- Alexis Powerblazer
- Susan Smartjacket
- Barbara Walters

Inner Feelings

It's around this time in the pregnancy where your wife will be able to feel the fetus move. Scott's wife described it as a sort of flutter, like a gas bubble deep in her belly. It is a fact that your wife, in her excitement, will tell you to put your hand on her stomach and try to feel the movement. It is also a fact that the world's most sensitive seismic equipment would fail to detect any activity in your wife's abdomen.

The Dudes suggest being honest about this (for now). You likely won't be called an insensitive jerk for not being able to feel your baby's movements at this point, as your wife won't be able to feel the movement with her own hand on her belly. The only reason we even bring it up is because she'll be certain to tell you about every undetectable flutter she feels from this point on. When she wakes you in the middle of the night to force you to not feel the baby moving, it will help prepare you for weeks down the road, when she wakes you in the middle of the night to feel the baby move (which you probably won't be able to feel).

Ask The Dudes

Dear Dudes,

I've been having A LOT of _anxiety_ lately about my wife's pregnancy. I'm starting to think that maybe I'm not the real father. What can I do to get over my fears? (yikes!)

AAAARGGHH!!

Sincerely,

Some Chump

write back soon! please !!!

Dear SC,

The only real option you have is the daytime talk show-brand paternity test. The Dudes advise you to practice your "That ain't my baby!" dance as much as possible. We've met your wife. There's a good chance you'll need it.

Sincerely,

The Dudes

Parental Advisory Warning

Once your wife is noticeably pregnant to others, she will face a barrage of unsolicited pregnancy advice from two types of people: old people and annoying people. Since

Science tells us that all old people are annoying, we can simplify: annoying people will give your wife pregnancy advice. She'll quickly learn to see it coming, though, and with practice might actually learn to avoid most of it. Normal people will give your wife a friendly I've-been-there-before smile and leave it at that, but your wife's protruding belly will be too tempting for the inherently irritating individual to ignore.

"Too bad for her," you may be thinking, and you may be right. But beware, dude. When you and your wife are around annoying people, you also get to be the recipient of whatever advice or nuggets of wisdom they have to offer. The indigent and the idiotic will cackle through their yellowed teeth or homemade holiday sweatshirts and tell you things that have nothing to do with anything, like

- "The more weight you gain, the happier the baby."
- "A baby gets a better night's sleep on its stomach."
- "Babies love cats, and cats love babies!"
- "Discipline starts in the delivery room."

One subcategory of aggravating advice-givers is the Great Big Fat Person. Great Big Fat People usually have something to say regardless of the situation. When spotting a pregnant woman, they tend to give unwanted advice in the form of anecdotes about their great big fat children, like, "When Francis was a little baby, he used to love a spoonful of peanut butter before bed." Really, chubs? Thanks for the lifesaving child-rearing tip.

The Dudes think it is safe to say you will receive absolutely no useful information from these people, unless they're telling you which denture adhesive works best or where to get the tastiest cheese fries in town.

🦢 Awesome Dudes' Observation 🦢

At some point during your wife's pregnancy, you are bound to hear someone gushing fondly about how you'll soon get to "meet" your new baby. Won't it be great when you finally get to "meet" your new son? The Dudes call bullshit on this. We call bullshit because you won't actually get to meet your son until he's twenty-eight years old and has finally stopped hating you and realized that you were actually right about a few things. Instead of saying "meet," The Dudes prefer "deal with." Won't it be great when you finally get to deal with your new son?

Midterms

Right around the midpoint of your wife's pregnancy, she'll be given a barrage of tests, some compulsory, some optional. The list includes

- *gestational diabetes.* Many women have a temporary bout of diabetes during pregnancy. A positive test simply means a little more attention to her diet, and it almost always goes away after delivery.
- *alpha-fetoprotein test.* It's a simple blood test to detect spinal abnormalities. Optional.
- *amniocentesis.* This one's got "awful" written all over it. The test for genetic defects involves drawing amniotic fluid through a syringe stuck into your

wife's belly and makes us think of the overdose scene in *Pulp Fiction,* only less funny.

Bill's wife experienced thirty-five minutes of hell in the emergency room while having a simple procedure performed, dubbed the Stupid Nurse Test. His wife was experiencing some bleeding at about five months, so they decided to take a late-night, better-safe-than-sorry trip to the emergency room. After several minutes of an ER nurse (aka glorified cleaning lady) searching for the fetal heartbeat, she decided to seek the help of a person with minimal medical training. While Bill and his wife waited a half an hour for said trainee, he tried to come up with some words to say to his wife when it was inevitably announced that she had lost the baby.

Since the ER doctor was too busy cleaning poo off an old lady, an actual OB nurse was tracked down and was able to quickly find the baby's steady heartbeat by placing the monitor on Bill's wife's lower belly (not on her head, as attempted by the ER nurse). Everything was fine.

These are just a few of the awful tests that will cause you and your wife extreme bursts of anxiety for the duration of the pregnancy.

Finger "DIC"-ing Good

Whenever Foreign Guy discovered a gadget, food, or animal that they didn't have in his country, he naturally assumed that he had to inform everyone that it existed. Such an opportunity arose once, when he heard Scott talking on the phone to his wife. Scott's wife was asking him to pick up some frosted cookies and fifty cans of apricot juice. When Scott got off the phone, Foreign Guy leaned over the cubicle wall with some advice. "Do you know of this place called KFC? I say that it is magnificent. Your wife would enjoy very much this place. They have extra large sampler bucket for fried chicken. The selection for side dishes have many choices and you are allotted a half gallon of soft drink of your choice!"

Scott nodded and tried to look impressed.

"What contemporary American woman for not like fried chicken?" Foreign Guy then asked excitedly. Scott told him that he'd go home and take his wife out that same night. What Scott didn't have the heart to tell Foreign Guy was that he had already suggested fried chicken to his wife a couple of weeks ago. She reacted by quietly gagging and puking in her own mouth a little. Scott was forbidden from even mentioning fried chicken after that.

Myth vs. Fact

Myth: A unique name for your child will help him or her develop a sense of individuality.

Fact: A unique name for your child will help him get his candy ass kicked in school.

Myth: The elderly have invaluable advice for young families.

Fact: The elderly have nonvaluable advice for you, and they smell like mentholated ointment.

Myth: Not knowing the baby's gender can help your wife's motivation during delivery.

Fact: Not knowing the baby's gender can cost you loads of cash.

CHAPTER SIX

Weeks 23–26

It's official. Time to take it to the next level! As The Dudes are always looking for opportunities to take it to the next level, we were very excited about month six. What does the next level have in store for you? Well, if you're a fan of growing anxiety and insecurity, unwieldy breasts, stretch marks, and hemorrhoids, you'll definitely be in your glory, especially because your wife may be experiencing the same things in the coming weeks. A two-fer! Next level, here we come!

Cache Register

The Dudes have always thought that registering for gifts—wedding, baby, or otherwise—is a little bit pompous, kind of like saying, "You will buy us gifts, and here's what those gifts will be! In fact, here's a printed list of said gifts so you don't screw it up, dumbass!" Nevertheless, the concept does work quite nicely.

Like Bill, you can try to convince your wife to register for her baby shower at Home Depot or Pizza Hut. But, like Bill, you will fail. We know what you're thinking: "All that flooring and/or Meat Lover's pizza would be great!" This will not be the first or last time in her pregnancy, however, that your wife will be totally unreasonable. You will probably register at Babies "R" Us or some other meatless baby mecca.

When you do set out to tell people what to buy you via registering, expect to spend three to four hours in an above-mentioned meatless baby mecca. When you arrive, you'll get a scanner and possibly a list of suggested baby essentials. This will, of course, be in addition to the list that your wife has already created. The Dudes remind you that strategy is crucial here—a little strategy will help guarantee that you'll be gifted the most expensive items instead of having to pay for a $300 stroller out of your own pocket. You can then pass the savings on to yourself and indulge in the aforementioned large deep-dish pizza after your registering ordeal.

Register for all the expensive stuff first. People want to buy cool things for you. Don't register for lame token gifts just because you're worried the other cool stuff might be a bit pricey. Your gift-giving friends and family will often pool resources to buy you the more expensive gifts on your list. Bill's wife had a second shower for out-of-state relatives a couple months after her first big shower. All that was left on the registry were dozens of smaller, yet still essential, items. Friends and family do not want to buy nipple balm, hemorrhoid pillows, or Episiotom-Ease, unless that friend/family member is a pervert and wants to store the thought of your wife using these items. If the registry is well picked over by the time your rich aunt Penelope gets around to having "the help" purchase a gift for you, she may take it upon herself to buy something she thinks is adorable. But we all know Aunt Penelope is freakin' crazy. Seriously, the lady paints on her damn eyebrows, for Christ's sake. She's rich, though…and that's why we love her. It would be a shame to have her squander her riches on something like mint green bibs that say "Spit Happens" (and if you think that's funny, then you're part of the problem).

Remember: register for stuff that females think is cute. Don't clog the registry with items that will force people to spend their money on stuff that you can pick up yourself for a few bucks. It's better to buy the aforementioned few-buck items yourself than to have to spend $250 on a crib mattress. By not giving people other options, you're forcing them to buy you the cool, expensive stuff. Plus, you can rest better knowing that you've put one over on them. That is, unless they haven't had kids yet, in which case you're setting yourself up to get screwed in kind when it's their turn to procreate. Good luck.

While your wife might think she knows what the baby will need, you do have some input in the registry process—input you should use as wisely as possible. The Dudes know that thinking ahead about your baby's registry needs is about as exciting as suffering through an episode of *A Baby Story* on television. So we've put together a helpful list of items that you (and your baby) might need and ways of justifying putting them on the baby registry.

■ Heavy-duty 36 V cordless reciprocating saw, to replace the one that your asshole "friend" Carl borrowed and sold to pay off his dealer. Tell your wife that you'll probably use it to help build something awesome for the baby someday.

■ Heavy-duty 9 HP 17-gallon gas wheeled portable air compressor. If your wife resists, simply tell her that by saying no, she'd be robbing your baby of the precious gift of [compressed] air. And what baby doesn't need [compressed] air?

■ Heavy-duty 3,750 PSI gas pressure washer with hose reel. If your wife would rather have a lame stroller, simply explain to her that you've heard that babies tend to make messes, and you're being proactive. She'll most likely give in when you elaborate on how 3,750 pounds per square inch of water pressure will pretty much clean the (baby) shit out of anything.

You might have to register at Home Depot or some similar tool fortress, but believe us when we tell you that you won't regret a thing when your wife tears open that pastel-colored baby shower wrapping paper and finds a beautiful new heavy-duty 1/2" (13 mm) 36 V cordless hammerdrill/drill/driver kit staring back at her.

At Your Disposal

The Dudes would like to take this opportunity to warn you, the potential baby product consumer, about a product on the market that people might try recommending to you. The product is essentially a diaper pail with a "sealed" lid. It's a smallish, plastic-lined garbage can that you can use to magically dispose of your baby's diapers. It employs a long, often scented, specially designed garbage bag and some sort of sealing lid. There are many similar products on the market as well.

Up front, it seems like a fantastic idea. Put the diaper in, twist the knob, and the diaper disappears into a pleasantly scented bag for all eternity. We love the idea; it's fantastic. In practice, though, it's not exactly like that. These products remind us of razors or computer printers. The companies will almost give you the razor handle or printer for free.

However, they will then proceed to stab you in the balls with the cost of razor blades and ink cartridges.

Proving that the printer and razor companies don't have a monopoly on ball-stabbing, you'll get the same deal with one of these high-tech diaper pails. The can is cheap; the refills are not. Plus, every different brand has its own bags to sell, and it's hard to tell which stores carry which brands.

On top of all of that, the thing only works half the time. Eventually the baby-poo odor magically becomes one with the plastic of the can. Science tells us that once plastic fuses with poo (see diagram below), the only option you have is to throw the whole deal away. It just reeks that bad after time, despite those special bags you're forced to buy.

The Dudes have found that the best solution to the diaper disposal problem is to use all those plastic bags you get from the grocery store. In fact, start saving them today. By the time your baby is born, you'll have an ample stockpile to handle even the worst diapers. Simply bag it and toss it in the outside garbage can immediately.

So, no matter what people say, don't put this thing on your registry. Find some other useless but nonstinky baby item instead.

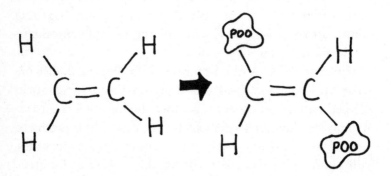

Gene Pool Party

A baby shower consists of a group of women—each trying to look cuter than the next—gathering for the purpose of ooh-ing, ahh-ing, and even applauding very small clothes.

This is an actual quotation from Bill's wife in the days leading up to the baby shower:

Wife: "I can't wait for my show...umm, I mean our show...umm, I mean the baby's shower!"

The shower is generally a very good thing, though, since it involves people giving you free baby-oriented gifts, some of which you actually need. Bill was personally very happy to haul home a swing, playpen, baby monitor, and diapers, not to mention enough clothing to dress a small country (of babies). After some calculations, he figured that the baby would have to wear four to five different outfits daily in order to actually wear all the clothes she got before she outgrew them...which is, of course, exactly the plan (see page 125, which discusses the baby being a doll for grown-up girls).

If you're lucky, the host of the shower will not have planned a "couples shower," in which case you can show up at the end, say hi to Grandma, pack up your stuff, grab a few leftover deviled eggs, and hit the road. On the other hand, if you are forced to endure the dreaded couples shower, your wife's friends will bring husbands or dates, and all the guys get to punch you in the nuts as they leave. Please note that the punching will be ten times worse if your mother-in-law made them play stupid baby-shower games.

While not all dudes will go through the horror of the couples shower, we thought it fitting to warn you about what to expect if your mother-in-law or, as in Scott's unfortunate case, your mother, actually plans this particular type of nightmare for you.

When your friends arrive at the couples shower bearing gifts, it is likely that most of the guys will have no clue what is in store for them. They might be a bit surly for having been dragged to the event in the first place, but they won't totally hate you. Yet. The hatred comes when the games begin.

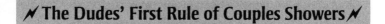

✒ The Dudes' First Rule of Couples Showers ✒

**Each heterosexual male at a couples shower
will contemplate suicide at least once
during said couples shower.**

The above rule is almost always a direct result of being subjected to one or more of the following baby-shower games—games, we might add, that women find exactly as funny as men don't find them funny. At all.

■ Guess the baby: Each person is required to bring a baby picture of himself or herself. Hilarity does not ensue as the guests try to match up the cute baby to the ugly adult.

■ Diaper candy-bar game: A chocolate, turd-shaped candy bar is slightly melted onto a baby diaper by your sinister mother or mother-in-law. Hilarity does not ensue as the women try to get the men to eat it.

■ Baby-food blindfold game: Quite possibly the most evil game ever invented. The women blindfold the men, then spoon-feed them random baby food and ask them to guess what it was they just ate. Hilarity does not ensue as the male guests begin to spit, gag, and dry heave while the women laugh at them. Most of Scott's friends still hate him to this very day because of this horrible game. (Note from Bill: I still hate you, Scott.)

The Dudes advise you to do anything in your power to prevent the couples baby shower. Seriously. Anything.

The Rite Stuff

As you will soon discover, your baby needs a great many things, things you might never have expected a baby to need. Aside from the standard stuff, like diapers, milk, and TV, you might be surprised to learn that your baby will cry if it does not have several of the following:

- A new house—the old one is just not fit for raising a child in.
- A new car—because pregnancy will, somehow, suddenly make your old "new car" incredibly unsafe.
- An entire room of your home, complete with new paint job and baby theme.
- A crib, changing table, rocking chair, toy box, bassinet, swing, and noisy bouncy jumpy thing.
- A new, expensive digital camera and video recorder.
- A new paint job in the living room, kitchen, your bedroom, and pretty much every other room that the baby might happen to be in someday.

You'll also be surprised to find out that your baby will *need* these things *before* it is born. Yep, that's right: Before. It. Is. Born. "But how can this be?" you might be asking yourself and anyone else who will listen. Well, since your baby can't directly communicate its dislike of unsafe cars and old paint to the outside world, you'll have to use the built-in interpreter, its mother. That's right, your wife is your direct line of communication to your baby, and she will tell you often that it's not *she* who needs these things, but the baby. *Your* baby. How could you deny your baby the very things—as relayed to you by its mother—it needs to survive?

After the "it's your baby, not me" card has been played, you pretty much have no choice. Who wants a sad baby on his conscience forever? Yes, *forever*—even if that baby is still tucked away in your wife's guts somewhere. It's best to try to just go along with the more reasonable demands. Mothers have an innate ability to convince you to convince yourself that you actually *do* need this stuff... all of it. After all, it's for your baby, right? Pretty soon, you might actually believe that you need a ridiculously expensive, gas-guzzling SUV and 8,000-square-foot house—for the baby. And while it is true that when a baby is born, it can hardly see, barely move, and only wants to eat and sleep, everything *must* be in place, from the unoccupied-for-months-to-come crib to the unusable two-piece baby bikini. "A place for everything, and everything in its place" seems to be the motto of choice during this troubling phase.

For those men who might be having a hard time grasping the absurdity of this, think about what happens when you put a brand-new tool in your toolbox. You experience an almost uncontrollable urge to organize the entire toolbox to accommodate the new tool. Or how about when you get a new car and feel the urge to clean the garage... or carport... or car hole, or whatever. Anyway, it's the same thing with pregnant women, except that the tool is the baby, the toolbox is your life, and organizing it will require all of your money and spare time, and a modest portion of your sanity.

Changing Room

The baby wants *everything* to be *perfect* for its arrival. If you don't believe that, watch as your six-months-pregnant wife polishes the forks four to six times a day, regardless of the fact that—aside from jamming them into electrical outlets—infants seldom have use for eating utensils.

In an effort to please your unborn child, your wife will insist that the baby's room (nursery) is fully functional—and more important, awe-inspiringly adorable—several months before its arrival. This will include some sort of theme painting, wallpapering, and stocking with toys, clothes, a mobile, and cute baby furniture. This cute furniture includes, but is not limited to, a changing table, dresser, and crib/mattress/bedding set. Sure, any dresser can double as a changing table, but that doesn't matter. Sure, the baby will be sleeping in amniotic fluid for a few more months, but that doesn't matter either, because the baby wants these things, and thankfully your wife has been contracted to see that it gets them.

Oh, and to further twist the dagger of irony, your wife will demand that the baby sleep in a bassinet beside your bed for several months after its birth, ensuring your laboriously crafted nursery remains a life-size infant diorama for months to come.

Equipping the nursery is one of the joys of pregnancy for women. Searching for the perfect furniture for her will be like looking through the toy section of the Sears Christmas catalog used to be for you. At least until you discovered the boobs in the lingerie section, a discovery that was likely followed by you wondering how they manage to find so many hot, nippleless models.

When she finally does settle on the perfect furniture, there is a 95 percent chance that you'll have to order it. It is important to note here that there is a 100 percent chance that your order will get completely fucked up somewhere along the way. It doesn't matter if you placed the order or not, it will be your fault, and you will probably have to call and get the whole thing straightened out. If she does the calling, we seriously feel sorry for the poor bastard on the other end.

We tell you this in order to avert an even bigger disaster that's looming on the horizon—the possibility that the furniture won't arrive until *after* the baby has. While this would technically not be a problem for the baby, it will be for your wife. Scott once witnessed a pregnant coworker call about a screwed-up crib order. In the middle of a crowded office, this woman was literally screaming at the guy on the phone, sarcastically asking him where the hell the baby was going to sleep once it was born. Any guy with kids would have just told here that her baby could sleep peacefully in the bassinet (for months) until the crib arrived. Apparently, though, the guy didn't have kids, and she'd reduced him to a gibbering wuss by the end of her tirade.

As you can see, this furniture is something that you should probably take a little more seriously than your brain foolishly tells you to. It's just one less thing for you to worry about in a future filled with you worrying about a bunch of other crap. Crap like forcing your religion, politics, and sexuality on your future fighter pilot.

While we're on the subject, we'd like to add a bit more

about the changing table. Don't be so foolish as to think you can just use an ordinary dresser as a changing table. You can't. We don't know why, but you just can't. It's like quantum physics. The more you try to understand it, the more you want to stop trying to understand it.

The changing table is simply a dresser with a raised end containing a drawer. This drawer houses all of the baby maintenance equipment. Think of it as the baby toolkit: diapers, lotions, wipes, powders, creams, and anything else used to de-funk your baby. Why this equipment needs its own drawer is part of the eternal mystery that we happily defer to anyone else but us to figure out.

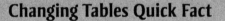

✓   **Changing Tables Quick Fact**   ✓

While any changing table can easily become
a dresser, the reverse is never true.

Bassinet Instincts

When you were a young boy staging elaborate scenes with your Star Wars figures so you could douse them with lighter fluid and burn them to the ground ("This is for what you did to Luke, Jabba!"), your future wife was meticulously dressing a variety of dolls in a variety of outfits and foolishly not setting them on fire. As a result, you are now prepared to destroy any sebaceous alien crime boss you may encounter at the local Sarlac-pit, and your wife is prepared to dress your newborn child in a variety of cute outfits. Your wife will spend the remainder of her pregnancy sitting in the meticulously crafted nursery for six to twelve hours a day going through all the clothes she got at the shower, perhaps laying out baby clothes in the order they will be forcibly tried on.

Bill's wife had a special way of preparing for the baby's arrival. She determined that on her first day home, she would begin the outfit rotations, taking pictures of the baby in each outfit to send to the person who had given the outfit at the shower. She of course had each of the hundred or so outfit/giver-of-outfit combos in her mental Rolodex and could recall the pairing with retarded genius–like proficiency. The onesie with the turtle on it with a pocket: her mom. The onesie with the turtle on it, no pocket: Bill's mom.

You may eventually notice during the costume changes to come that the more useless the outfit is, the cuter it is. Example: a white onesie is practical, useful, comfy, and easy to put on and remove. It rates somewhere between not cute and marginally cute. The baby two-piece bikini, however, is impractical, difficult to put on, and probably dangerous. Nonetheless, it is infinitely adorable.

Outer Feelings

After weeks and weeks of pretending that you can feel the baby move, the time has finally come when you don't have to fake it anymore. You can now share the creepy joy that comes from feeling the baby kicking and jabbing at your wife's internal organs. This might come with a sense of relief to you, because it's confirmation that there's actually something other than your wife's imagination growing in there.

During this time, the baby will try to pick fights with any of your wife's internal organs that make the mistake of looking at it wrong. This is perfectly normal, and it's not unusual to see your wife suddenly jump out of her seat and yell at her belly in an accusatory tone. She probably just got kicked in the ribs, so don't be alarmed.

Although the baby is only six months old, its archnemesis is often your wife's bladder. Every time her bladder makes the mistake of getting full, your baby will feel obligated to start a no-holds-barred street fight with it. Eventually your wife will be forced to run to the bathroom so her bladder can concede defeat. Whether or not she makes it to the bathroom is of no consequence to your triumphant baby.

ⓘ   **Not So Fun Fact**   ⓘ

Some people think that drinking a pregnant woman's urine will give them superimmunity to disease and prolong their lives. The Dudes think that "some people" are batshit crazy.

Full Belly

Your wife's cute little baby belly is fast becoming a thing of the past. Make way for the newer, more-stretched-out version. The full-on one-in-the-oven belly is finally making its appearance. This is usually cause for great concern amongst men, and if you're feeling some anxiety, consider yourself perfectly normal. As you know, The Dudes always give you the nonwussified, nonsugarcoated truth. It's now time to face the music, boys—your wife's hot, flat, nonstretchy belly is gone, and without serious effort, most likely gone forever. It's okay to cry if you want to; we totally understand. Just do it where she can't hear you.

One of the strange things you might encounter during the rest of your wife's pregnancy is the irresistible urge of strangers to reach out and touch her belly. This is sometimes an older woman, but not always. Try not to be too alarmed when the old woman at the grocery store suddenly reaches out and pokes your wife in the gut. This is often followed by her mumbling something about the kids that abandoned her years ago, only to call monthly to make sure she hasn't spent all of their inheritance.

Tan Line

Another exiting way that Nature has of screwing with your wife's body is something called the linea nigra, or black line. This is a dark line on the skin that stretches from her crotch to her belly button, and often unmercifully continues up to the bottom of her ribs. This pregnancy gem sometimes includes coarse, dark hairs similar to what that guy in *The Fly* had to deal with right before he shot himself in the face. Our friend Science told us that it has something to do with hormones, but beyond that, he had no idea. While we didn't see this particular oddity on our wives, our friend Chuck assured us that it is indeed a reality. He even offered to take pictures to prove it. We politely declined.

Dr. Dude Says

"Pregnancy hormones can cause increased hair growth on the abdomen, face, arms, or elsewhere. Conversely, hair loss after delivery isn't uncommon. Freakin' hilarious, huh?"

Breasts Redux

At this point, The Dudes would like to congratulate you on your wife's enormous juggs. We're just the first, though. Expect congratulations from any male over the age of twelve with the gift of eyesight. Like all the upsides of pregnancy, however, you are about to have the downside shoved into your glaring face. "The Girls" are about to take on a life of their own and then turn completely gross. The eye candy that you've enjoyed over the last few months will quickly start to resemble evil aliens from a low-budget horror flick. The expanding masses won't stab you in the base of the neck and inject you with their mind-controlling offspring, but they will swell to the point of being translucent and veiny. They will become the consistency of pizza dough (thin crust) and will be about as much fun to play with...yeah, like you'd be allowed to anyway.

Likewise, just when you think the nipples have completed their scary size and color transformation, they present to you the gift of Montgomery Glands. If you're a regular reader of *Hustler* magazine or a frequent visitor to strip clubs with no cover charge, you've probably seen Montgomery Glands before. Your wife will likely be blessed with these rings of areola bumps circumnavigating her nipples. If she's extra lucky, she'll get the gift of an oily secretion from said glands. And if she's superlucky, she, like most women, will have these bumps for the rest of her life.

On the bright side, that's the last of the pregnancy surprises for boobs. It's the last time we'll even mention them until our next book, *The Dudes' Guide to Living with Your Wife's Shriveled Boobs That Are Now Smaller Than Before She Got Pregnant* (Wellness Central, 2009).

Permanent Markers

It's at this time when pregnancy potentially bestows upon your wife, and thus you, the gift of stretch marks, those purple lines that loud women with dudes' haircuts say "real women" have. We say "potentially" because there's a chance your wife won't get any stretch marks. So how does one avoid them then? Being careful not to gain too much weight? Using expensive stretch mark–prevention creams? A couple extra "audits" a week down at the Scientology center? Sorry, but none of these help. Neither proper diet, pricey salves, nor the powerful late L. Ron Hubbard can save you now.

Stretch marks are purely hereditary. For those of you unfamiliar with the concept, "hereditary" basically means that there's not a goddamn thing you can do about it. Science tells us that if her mother got stretch marks from carrying your wife or her siblings, they will likely blossom on your wife's belly as well. Science also tells us that if her mom didn't get stretch marks, there's a chance your wife may get them anyway. Science does this because he is a complete asshole.

Private DIC

Scott's DIC coworker Bitter Divorce Guy loves to tell the story of his wife's pregnancy and his search for stretch marks. Knowing that stretch marks were linked to genetics, Bitter Divorce Guy figured the best way to see if his wife was going to be "ruined" was to give his mother-in-law the once-over. Although The Dudes hardly endorse his plan, it seemed to get the desired result, that result being Foreign Guy throwing up in his mouth a little.

"I tell you what," Bitter Divorce Guy started, "I ain't never getting married again after seeing that shit." His plan involved "accidentally" walking in the bathroom after his visiting mother-in-law's morning shower.

"I walk in to see her toweling off, and I swear to God, the old broad had gray pubes," he said, making Scott recoil in terror.

"Why didn't you just ask your wife?" interrupted Sensitive Guy.

"Why don't you go fuck yourself? Anyway, all I could think about was, you know that scene in *The Shining* where that old lady gets out of the tub and the guy starts making out with her, and shit? I couldn't get that image out of my head for weeks, end of story."

A few awkward seconds later, Scott asked, "So did you ever find out?"

"Find out what?" said Bitter Divorce Guy.

"Jesus, if she had stretch marks!?" Scott said impatiently.

"Oh, yeah. I dunno. She was too wrinkly to tell. But I do know that my wife got some stretch marks, and I'll tell you, that was the beginning of the end."

Another semivaluable lesson learned, thanks to The Dudes in Cubes.

📖 Myth vs. Fact 📖

Myth: Using special lotions is the best way to avoid getting stretch marks.

Fact: Not getting pregnant is the best way to avoid getting stretch marks.

Myth: Only approved baby-changing dressers should be used to change your baby's diaper.
Fact: Outdoor babies don't require diapers at all.

Myth: Hiring a baby-shower planner is a good idea.
Fact: Hiring a baby-shower stripper is a fucking great idea.

CHAPTER SEVEN

Weeks 27–30

Welcome to the third trimester. If all hell breaks loose and your wife's body decides it's time to have a baby, odds are very good your little 3- to 4-pounder will be just fine. The significance of this for you is realizing that you've got a real, live, honest-to-God human in there now. And the aching, swelling, water retention, and general awkwardness is a constant reminder to you and your wife (who may also exhibit the symptoms listed).

Labor Intensive

Should you choose to accept the challenge, you will be attending some sort of class to teach you about labor and delivery. Scott and his wife—well, mainly just his wife—chose to get it all done in one weekend in a two-day, ten-hour workshop, leaving Scott feeling like he was in some sort of *Breakfast Club*–like parallel pregnant universe. He even fantasized about breaking out of there through the air ducts, Judd Nelson–style, all the while totally rockin' out to Wang Chung's "Fire in the Twilight" and crying about getting his butt cheeks taped together in gym class while screaming, "I'M SORRY, DAD! I'M SO SORRY!!"

Suffice it to say there was no crusty old principal, no essays to write, and relatively little teen angst. Well, except, for the knocked-up teenage girl who was there with her mother who Scott thought kinda looked like Ally Sheedy. A once-per-week class is more common than a weekend baby-class marathon and will probably bring you back to the glory days of when you got your GED (damn, those were some good times, weren't they?).

Baby class is a lot like high school, except that if in high school they'd showed us videos of naked chicks—well, minus the birthing parts, anyway—we probably would have enjoyed it a lot more. We also would have enjoyed it more if the film wasn't made in 1974, back before razors were invented. The irony, however, was the awfulness that these women were going through, and thus the anguish we experienced by watching them go through it (through the spaces between our fingers). Yes, if you haven't seen one before, you will see your first snuff film in a prenatal education class. You will also discover that there are some things you simply can't un-see, no matter how hard you try.

Of course, the whole premise of these classes is to shock you in order to prepare you for the real thing. The videos actually aren't that much worse than what you might see on the Oprah channel on any given Saturday morning. What you want to watch out for are slides, which Scott's instructor kept up long enough (two to three minutes each) so that the images could be burned into his head permanently. If you're lucky, one of the close-up slides might show you the heart-rate monitor they might *screw* into your unborn child's head. We wish we were making that up.

| 📢 | **Helpful Advice** | 📣 |

No matter how hilarious you think you are, never
jokingly refer to the childbirth process as "crapping
out a kid," especially when your wife is within earshot.
The reasons for this should be obvious, but if they aren't,
go ahead and give it a try.

Tackling Fundamentals

Your baby classes will probably be pretty boring. Some of
them you might actually find useful, like the one on infant
CPR, or the one on how to suppress your gag reflex while
changing your baby's crap-laden diaper. The class we feel
the need to specifically warn you about, though, is the one
on labor and delivery.

In this class, the instructor will probably refer to you as
"Labor Coach," "Coach Dad," or some other ridiculous,
patronizing crap. They do this in hopes of making you feel
like Mr. Awesome just for being there. Maybe they're playing off your lifelong semiurge to be an NFL head coach or
something. The truth of the matter is that they just think
it's "cute" that you're there with your wife. Furthermore,
if you weren't there, they'd look upon your wife with pity,
wondering why the biological father was out buying crack
and not sitting next to his baby's mamma enjoying the
novelty of being called coach. You'll get a strange feeling
when you're there. It's an overwhelming feeling that the
girls are all in on the joke, and you're left swingin' free
without your jock, just like in high school gym class. That
feeling won't be misplaced, either. Not by a long shot.

We're going to let you in on the secret, so at least you'll know why they're silently laughing at you. The secret is this: in the modern delivery room, there is absolutely no real reason why you should be there. There is nothing you can do to really help. There is nothing you can say to change anything. No matter how many ice chips you shove into your grunting wife's mouth, it won't matter. The doctors and nurses will do everything for you, relegating you to the sidelines as a glorified water boy. Ironically, there will be a large, screaming naked woman on a table soiling herself with a variety of fluids and solids for several straight hours, and *you'll* be the annoying one in the room. Sit quietly in the corner, out of everyone's way, and you'll be accused of not being helpful. Run around the delivery room urinating on everything, and all of a sudden, you're the crazy guy.

Don't think we're complaining, though. After all, they're the ones with the rubber gloves and face shields. We simply want to help you avoid any delusions of grandeur regarding your role in all this, because baby class is only a scam to make you feel better. It's a scam to make you think that aside from providing the sperm in the beginning, you actually matter in the delivery room. The class is designed this way on purpose in order to guarantee you'll show up to help fill out insurance paperwork and fetch ice. It seems to work quite well, too.

Knowing that, you'll now be able to at least awkwardly pretend like you're supporting your wife when that day finally arrives, even though all you'll be doing to help is exactly nothing. As you can imagine, providing this imaginary support will have its advantages three months down the road, when you finally get to score again.

Free, for All

One of the benefits of baby class is the free crap they give out. Companies will give loads of product samples to the hospitals that teach these classes to get you hooked, much like the local crack dealer. After the free stuff runs out, you're forced to buy more. That's how they getcha—again, like the local crack dealer. One way to prolong the initial high is to do what our friend John did.

After his class, John noticed that people were being polite and only taking one or two diapers each. He also noticed that there were enough diapers to fill a large garbage bag. Realizing the amazing opportunity, John calmly waited for his classmates to clear out of the room for their tour of the hospital. With ninjalike stealth, he ducked back into the room and closed the door. He grabbed an empty garbage bag from the can and stuffed as many free diapers into it as he could, cramming it full faster than a fat lady at a butter-eating contest. He then caught up with the group, carrying with him his well-deserved garbage bag full of free diapers. John's is just another example of what it takes to be a good father.

List of Fun Questions to Ask in Baby Class

You might be tempted to ask serious-sounding questions in baby class. You might do this to make all the other women in the room think you care. We admit it. It feels good. But it also feels good to get the truth out in the open. With that in mind, we've devised the following list of fun questions you might want to ask while in baby class. For maximum effectiveness (sarcasm), use the most sincere-sounding voice you can muster.

- Can I stay after class to review some more film?
- After the baby is born, should I be embarrassed by my tears of joy?
- During delivery, how often should I lovingly dab my wife's forehead with a cool, damp cloth?
- Would anyone mind if I took up a donation after class for the unfortunate girl (point at girl) who came with her mother?

and finally...

- How upset should I be that I will never get to experience vaginal delivery?

Rub Her Soul

One of the things your wife will undoubtedly experience during the remainder of her pregnancy is swelling of the extremities. We're not exactly sure why it's necessary for her to gain 40 pounds of water weight in each ankle; it just is. We tried to ask Science, but every time he tried to look, his eyes got watery and his gag reflex kicked in.

The swelling causes irritation and soreness and can be partially remedied by massage. At first it will seem impractical to hire a professional therapist to come into your home to massage your wife's feet and hands. Over time, you might start to consider it. Till then, though, the job falls to you.

Try to imagine massaging a flesh-covered, overfilled water balloon. Now, try to imagine massaging said water balloon as the person whose leg it's attached to is grunting and groaning and telling you how great it's going to feel when you do the other foot, too. Can't wait, can you?

There are special techniques to be used on the feet and

hands, so don't think you can use the prepregnancy massage know-how that you learned from your dirty college girl-friend. In one of Scott's baby classes, the "instructor" called her method of massaging hands "breaking the Popsicle." Scott was supposed to imagine that his wife's hand was one of those Popsicles with two sticks and then massage her hand using the same technique you'd use to "break the Popsicle." Scott wasn't prepared for the number of times he'd actually hear his wife say, "Honey, will you break my Popsicle?"

The Dudes advise you to prepare your hands for this strenuous work in advance. If you're going to do the massage, get one of those hand-gripper things and give your hands a workout. If you're going to half-ass the massage (our recommended approach), then just pretend to use it. Getting a hand cramp while massaging your wife's bloated feet can be really painful and a great excuse for you to stop doing it. It's always best to stop a hand cramp before it even gets started, and this can be accomplished by limiting your massage time to about forty-five seconds per extremity. That way you can technically say that you gave her the massage, and she can't tell her sister and/or friends that you didn't.

Giving her a massage might not seem like a big deal now, but picture yourself doing it a couple of times a day for the next three months. And hey, once you've started, she'll see no reason why the practice can't continue well after your child is born. We're just trying to help, is all.

An important issue that this whole massage business raises is that of your wife telling her mom/sister/friends anything/everything that you did/didn't do for/to her while she was/is pregnant. It's going to happen, so the best you can do is try to limit the fallout. Try to take away her ammo every chance you get, like with the aforementioned forty-five-second massages.

DICs: 'Rrhoid Rage

After a weekend of baby class, Scott returned to work better prepared to sift through the mountains of pregnancy advice heaped on him by his coworkers. Armed with infant CPR techniques and lifesaving diaper-changing procedures, he was prepared for the inevitable, "So, what did you do over the weekend?" from Sensitive Guy.

When it happened, Scott casually said, "Oh, nuthin', just went to baby class is all…" Upon hearing that, Sensitive Guy started talking about all the awesome stuff that he learned in his pregnancy classes and about how much he enjoyed actually applying the knowledge. He talked about how nice all the women in class were and about how he felt sorry for the girl who showed up with her mom.

As he droned on and on, Bitter Divorce Guy stopped by to listen in. Interrupting Sensitive Guy midsentence, he said, "I gotta tell ya, I didn't learn shit in those baby classes." Pausing to think, he went on, "Come to think of it, that's probably because I never actually went to any of them."

Sensitive Guy didn't skip a beat, and ignoring Bitter Divorce Guy, he went on to relate one of the most horrific stories Scott had ever heard. He said that some time during the last few months of pregnancy, his wife had developed hemorrhoids. Scott had learned in baby class that this was a fairly common problem for pregnant women. Luckily, though, his wife had been spared so far. What was not common, however, was how Sensitive Guy handled the situation.

"She asked me to go to the store and get some special cream, so I did," said Sensitive Guy. Cringing, Scott had already had enough, but Sensitive Guy was on a roll at that point, and Scott couldn't find a way out of the conversation. Sensitive Guy continued, "When I got back home, she even asked me to apply it for her because her size was restricting her reach."

"Holy shit, no!!!" Scott's brain screamed at him, telling him to run away as fast as he could. If he had had a cyanide tooth, he wouldn't have hesitated to use it right then. He'd seen Sensitive Guy's wife when she wasn't pregnant, all 220 pounds of her. Imagining her pregnant made him shudder. He knew where this story was going, but like watching a train wreck, he was powerless to stop it.

Sensitive Guy mercilessly continued on. "Women have enough to go through with pregnancy, so of course I told her I'd help. I mean, can you think of a better way of bonding with your soul mate than helping alleviate some of her suffering?"

"Ew," was all Scott's brain could muster at that point.

Sensitive Guy: "I removed the cap from the tube and squirted out some cream to lubricate the applicator."
Scott's brain: "No, God."
Sensitive: "A little embarrassed, my wife smiled. I told her everything would be fine."
Brain: "Think of a happy place."
Sensitive: "Calmly, I asked my wife to spread her..."

Before he could continue, Bitter Divorce Guy interjected from over the cube wall, "You better end this story right fucking now, man. She made you do it because she didn't want to touch her own butt, end of story. And Christ, do you have to be so fucking detailed all the time? I tell you what, Scott, I ain't never getting married again, you can count on that."

Scott took that as his cue to get the hell out, and he did so as quickly as possible.

📖   Myth vs. Fact   📖

Myth: You will be a vital member of the delivery team as the "birth coach."
Fact: You will help the delivery along if you can manage to stay the fuck out of the way.

Myth: It's fun to meet pregnant couples in birth class who are sharing similar experiences.
Fact: It's surprisingly reassuring to see someone as huge as your wife in birth class.

Myth: Massaging your pregnant wife will give her physical and emotional comfort.
Fact: It is a scientific fact that babies hate massages. Who will be their advocate? WHO?!?

CHAPTER EIGHT

Weeks 31–35

Month eight brings with it several new *miracles* as you begin to see the light at the end of the birth canal. These include, but are not limited to, the miracles of poor leg circulation and varicose veins; the phenomenon of an itchy belly; the wonder of increased shortness of breath; the bounty of leaky nipples; and the manna-from-heaven–like, increased, heavy whiteish genital discharge. At this point in the game, your wife is almost certain to experience similar, if not the exact same, symptoms.

Snooze Alarm

It is no surprise at the eight-month mark that your wife will be tired all day long and unable to sleep when she finally goes to bed. Month eight often presents some especially cruel, sleep-depriving symptoms. Not only will she be miserable and unable to sleep, causing her to be tired throughout the following day yet unable to sleep the next night, but she will also take out the fact that she can't sleep on you, causing you not to sleep and making you sleepy throughout the following day, too. See where this is going?

First, the weight and center-of-gravity–distorting qualities of her abdomen make any sleep position ridiculously
uncomfortable...even painful. Your local fatty will be
able to easily explain—or perhaps show you—how difficult this is to live with. Fatty's explanation will probably
be given in exchange for some baked goods.

Women will invariably try sleeping with a pillow between their legs to offset something or another. This will
likely do no good because it all comes down to personal
comfort, which is hard to find for an eight-month-pregnant
chick.

Bill's wife bought a full body pillow, which she would
prop her protruding belly onto and wrap her legs around
while sleeping on her side. This seemed to keep her mostly
comfortable for the home stretch. As an added bonus, Bill's
wife kept the pregnancy pillow after the birth. It makes a
great divider down the center of the bed so she doesn't in-
vade his sleep space for spontaneous late-night snuggling.

Second, not having developed regular sleep habits yet,
the baby will relentlessly continue its attack of your wife's
ribs, guts, and bladder at night, causing her to wake up or
rush off to change her underwear, which she just peed in a
little. Merely getting out of bed can be a challenge. Imagine strapping a 40-pound weight to your belly and rolling around with it. Now stop imagining it, as you are not
pregnant and thus don't have to worry about such fantasti-
cal nonsense.

Finally, Science tells us that if your wife falls asleep on
her back, the weight of the baby will significantly cut off
the blood flow of a major artery to her legs, causing them
to "fall asleep." And although Science muttered something

about scoring some meth in the same sentence, we'll take him at his word on this one. We'd rather play it safe so as not to be awoken suddenly from our kick-ass dream of officiating the Lingerie Bowl by her barking orders to massage her legs back to working order before she pees the bed (again).

The Dudes Salute…

Dr. John Braxton Hicks, inventor of a hilarious way of fucking with your wife. In the early twentieth century, Dr. Braxton Hicks figured out a way to trick your wife (and thus you) into thinking that she's going into labor during the later months of pregnancy. His legacy lives on to this day. Behold as your wife's uterus contracts as if it's practicing for the big game. She'll have all the panic-inducing contractions of labor, minus the baby actually coming out of her vagina. Our hats off to you, John Braxton Hicks, M.D.

Very Ample Genitalia

If you love vaginas (and who doesn't?!?), what could be better than a *huge* VAGINA, you would think. The correct answer to this question is EVERYTHING. Everything is better than a huge vagina. Black jelly beans, ingrown toenails, female bloggers, parking tickets, leukemia, *Two and a Half Men*. These are all examples of things that are *way* better than a huge vagina. The only difference is the above-listed items won't be in your house every day during the last few months of your wife's pregnancy (and a few weeks after), unless there's a best of Charlie Sheen marathon on cable.

Of course, what good is enlarged vulva without its horrible sidekick, whiteish discharge (now with increased odor!)? Like a Hawaiian volcano god, your wife's V.A.G. is about to become angered and violently erupt, wreaking its vengeance upon the quivering Polynesians in its path. Coincidentally, this discharge resembles the baking soda/vinegar lava concoction from your grade-school science-fair project about volcanoes.

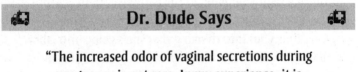

Dr. Dude Says

"The increased odor of vaginal secretions during pregnancy is not rare. In my experience, it is most common in western Pennsylvania."

Mixed Marital Arts

Although you may have had a brief sexual oasis in month four, you'll have noticed by months seven to nine how comically awkward sex has become. (Don't be surprised if it becomes uncomically nonexistent.) The expression "like a monkey humping a football" is useful in describing such relations. Only in this case, the football is 3 feet long and has a head and four limbs sticking out of it. Picture a scene you might see at the zoo, and after a few minutes wrestling with her, be content to resign yourself to beating your chest and masturbating.

Some men claim to really enjoy late-term-pregnancy sex

or even the mere idea of it. Through some form of crazy brain chemistry or DNA magic, they think it's the greatest thing ever. Maybe they dig it because it's dirty, or taboo, or feels like a very creepy three-way. Whatever the reason, it's definitely not our bag, and while we have yet to actually meet one of these guys in real life, we do know that they exist because the Internet tells us they do. Hell, there are entire Web sites devoted solely to pregnant women having sex. Let us not forget, though, that there are Web sites devoted to Japanese women eating puke, too. The Dudes subscribe to neither.

There's always some form of unpleasantness in store for you, no matter how beautiful those crappy shows on TLC that your wife forces you to watch tell you pregnancy is. Be sure to take quick mental snapshots of the hot girl at work, the girl with the thong sticking out at the gym, the girls in every beer commercial, etc. as the third trimester approaches, because you'll need to fortify your internal spank bank as much as possible, since you'll be making some significant withdrawals during that time.

Intercourse during the last months of pregnancy can best be summed up in one word: uncomfortablyfucking-awkward. Just accept it, like you accept that you're not one of those rare guys who actually gets turned on by it. Once you accept it, you can go about it like you do any other uncomfortable task. You can't stop having sex completely, or you'll run the risk of making her think that you think she's ugly or unattractive; after all, it's hard to tell your pregnant wife that it's nothing against her personally, but you're just not into pregnant chicks. So it's best not to even hint at it. In fact, your life will become even more of a living hell if you're stupid enough to actually tell her that. It's like the age-old question "Do these jeans make me look fat?" No, honey, they don't, now move your leg over there while I try to bend my raging semi around the bedpost.

The positioning alone is enough to make you give up in despair, sobbing and naked under the sweaty sheets. While we can offer little hope, we can offer some practical advice that will get you through this rough time. If you think you've got it all figured out, go knock yourself out. If not, let's get started with the (literally) gory details.

How about some good, old-fashioned missionary sex? Actually, that's a no go. As we just learned, when pregnant women lie on their backs, the child inside tends to rest right on top of some pretty important arteries. Cutting off the blood flow to the lower extremities is never a good thing and should probably be avoided as much as possible (unless, of course, you like seeing her legs turn blue and hearing her complain about dizziness).

But there are plenty of other positions, right? What about her on top? That usually results in you pushing in, and her pushing you right the hell back out. Also, the extra pregnancy pounds she's put on really come into play as they come crashing down on your unprepared pelvis. Not to mention that her baby-laden belly is right there in your face, causing you to think about your child more than you should while having sex.

Lots of those sex chapters in her pregnancy books will mention the nonmanly spooning position. Seriously, how many men actually enjoy the spooning position? Mostly it's done because it's a precursor to sex; it's hardly ever part of the actual sex itself. For good reason, too—because it sucks. You'd have to be Ron Jeremy to make this a really effective position, and since you're most likely not The Hedgehog, it's best to scratch this off the list right away.

Oh, but there's always oral, right? Yes, but during the late term, you'd have to be pretty brave to actually try this on her. The Dudes have one word for you here—discharge. Did you shudder when you read that? Get shivers up and down your back? Puke in your own mouth a little bit (again)? Well, congratulations, because that means you're perfectly normal.

Scott's neighbor once tried to describe the odor to him, and the best word he could come up with was "remarkable." Scott said, "Dude, that's all you need to say. I really don't want to hear any more." Thankfully, Scott's neighbor didn't want to think about it anymore either, and they both stood in front of the grill in awkward silence for the next five minutes.

You can try to get all fancy like they do in porn, but you'll probably find that in actual practice, those positions don't really work. The Dudes have compiled an incredibly helpful list of the most dangerous sexual positions to avoid during pregnancy.

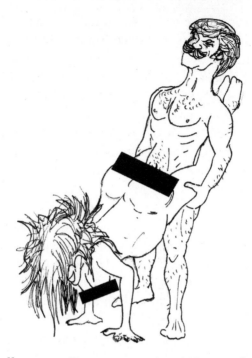

1. *Wheelbarrow*—Your once-petite, 110-pound wife now tips the scales just shy of huge. Not only will you have trouble getting a decent grip around her thighs, but she'll be forced to hold the push-up position. Remember, she'll have to hold it long enough for you to sift through your spank bank to find something powerful enough to overcome your tears. By the time that happens, her arms—along with your boner—will have completely given out. Avoid this demoralizing position at all costs.

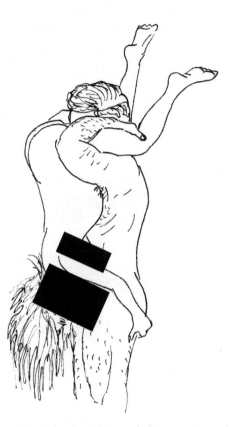

2. *Standing 69*—The logistics of this position have managed to completely baffle even our friend Science. That doesn't happen very often. If you can get past the idea of discharge and odor long enough to get a woody, you're not even close to being in the clear. Imagine the difficulty of lifting her high enough to achieve the proper angles. You'd have to construct some sort of pulley mechanism just to compensate for the added pressure on your quads alone. If you're looking to totally blast your quads, The Dudes recommend heading to the gym instead.

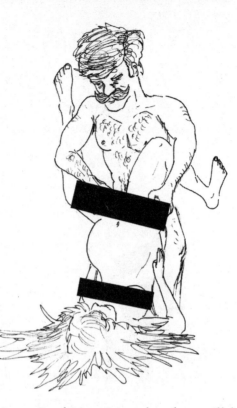

3. *Pile Driver*—In this position, her face will be totally blocked from view. At least that'll keep you from noticing how unbelievably fucking miserable she is. The Dudes recommend that if you actually try this, make sure you have a Magic Marker handy. Draw a smiley face on the underside of her belly to trick yourself into believing that she's actually having a good time.

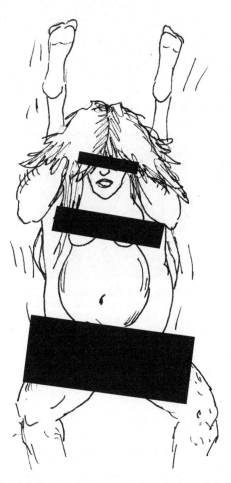

4. *Anal Full Nelson*—What would sex be without a heavy dose of professional wrestling? Hell, this acrobatic sexual position is even risky for completely nonpregnant gymnasts, let alone pear-shaped pregnant women with dangerously fucked-up centers of gravity. However, if you do actually manage to get her ankles behind her head, nature pretty much takes care of the rest.

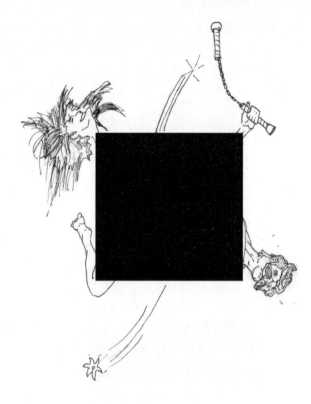

5. *Ninja's Revenge*—Whatever you do, Ninja's Revenge should never be considered an option for pregnancy sex. Not ever.

Go ahead and use your imagination if you want—try all the positions you can think of, but the results will always be the same: she'll be uncomfortable and complain of back pain, causing you to go limp with despair. Or maybe she'll tell you that she can feel the baby kick during the heavy pounding you think you're giving her, also causing you to go limp with despair. As you can see, it's going to be rough, and you'll mostly be limp and in despair.

The only two things we can suggest for making it work during this third trimester are a good, quick blowjob or doing it doggy-style. And though we know that it's hard to go wrong with a blowjob, it's definitely possible, so here are some of The Dudes' tips. Remember to always get some sort of pillow fort set up to block her belly from view, allowing you to suspend your belief long enough to enjoy the experience, but try to be quick about it. The irony here is that for years you probably tried to *increase* the duration of a blowjob, whereas now the goal is an efficiency that would make Stalin proud. Again, think of the children—by not thinking of the children.

If you choose the old, reliable doggy style, you'll have to remember that even though you aren't the above-mentioned Mr. Jeremy, in this position, you can still penetrate so deep, you can actually cause her pain. She might even complain that you're hurting the baby. So practice a little self-restraint in this position, stud, and you'll be rewarded with a view where, if you angle it just right, she might look only four months pregnant instead of eight. Push too hard, and you can actually induce some harmless bleeding, which will in turn induce a full night of utter panic. Good luck.

So there it is, the real, uncensored version of what to expect sexually during the third trimester. While we're sure this has all been very helpful to you, the future father, it has, more important, helped us exercise our demons.

ⓘ   Not So Fun Fact   ⓘ

Colostrum, or premilk, is produced by your wife's oversized boobs late in pregnancy. We're telling you this now because of the very real possibility of you losing your hard-earned erection by discovering it "on the job."

What Dreams May Come

The month of irony has more ironic plans to surprise you with...ironically. Turns out a lot of pregnant women's libidos kick into hyperdrive during the third trimester. This includes increased horniness, superintense orgasms, and an insatiable sex drive. Bill's wife would even occasionally wake up to orgasm in the middle of the night. That's right, a freaking *wet dream*. You remember those from junior high, don't you?

All of this of course flies in the face of everything we've told you/warned you about in this chapter. As is our style, The Dudes are merely laying out the facts here. How should you deal with it? We don't fucking know. Can't you figure out some shit on your own from time to time?!? Jeez! We guess we just remember a lot of crying in the fetal position and thinking of a happy place.

Dr. Dude Says

"In some cases, female orgasm has been found to bring on contractions in the later months of pregnancy. Because of this, The Dudes think it's best to concentrate only on what feels good for you. Don't give us any of that crap about her pleasure being stimulating to you, either. We're not buying it. It's *your* boner, not *hers*."

An Affair to Remember

Scott woke up one morning groggy—and hating his alarm clock—as usual. He snoozed the f'ing thing and closed his eyes. He tried to fall back asleep, but he couldn't. He had a nagging feeling that something was wrong. Very, very wrong. He lay there quietly, his sleepy head trying to piece together what was out of place, when suddenly he had one of those horror-movie moments. You know the kind, where the hot girl realizes that the killer is standing right behind her, about to plunge the chainsaw into her back. Except in this case, the hot girl was Scott, and the unstable chainsaw-wielding killer was his eight-months-pregnant wife. He finally realized that she had been quietly lying there, staring at him for at least half an hour, possibly all night, holding her chainsaw.

Scott cautiously turned to her to see what was wrong. Her cold, unblinking eyes were the first indication that he was totally screwed. What's worse is that he had no idea why. Before he could even say anything, she lashed out.

"Are you cheating on me?" she asked. Scott stared at her, never having even contemplated that question.

"Well?" she urged.

"What the hell are you tal—" he stammered in disbelief before she cut in, "Because I just had this dream."

Scott knew instantly that this was a battle he could not possibly win, so he just lay there and let her finish.

During pregnancy, women tend to have very vivid dreams involving a wide variety of horrible topics. Will the baby explode if I drop it? Will I eventually drive a mini-van? Is my husband cheating on me in real life because in my dream he was? The list goes on and on, but when your wife starts confusing her dreams with reality, you're in for some real trouble.

As with most of her issues during pregnancy, if this happens, it's best to just let her finish. She will eventually, hopefully, realize the insanity of her notion that you cheating in her dream means that you're cheating in real life (well, unless you really are cheating in real life, but that's a topic for an entirely different Dudes' guide—though probably one written by Scott's brother).

Anyway, being sleepy and sort of irritated, Scott said the worst thing he could have said at the time. He said, "Wait...so who was I banging, you know, in your dream?"

"Linda, from down the street," Scott's wife coldly replied. "You were *banging* Linda."

At hearing that, Scott was so offended that he couldn't do what he should have, which was to shut up and go to work. Linda, aka "Large Linda," was the stuff of nightmares.

"Linda!?" he shot back, "Oh, that's great! Why couldn't it have been an f'ing supermodel, or some famous actress, or even your sister!? What the hell!"

Then Scott's wife got all defensive, "Well, you were the one cheating. I can't help it if you chose Linda."

"I didn't choose her, it was *your* dream! How could you do that to me!?" He carried on as he got up. His brain was still trying to deal with the fact that he was having a real-world argument about doing neighbor Linda in *his wife's* dream.

Scott shook his head and tried to block it all out. "Screw this," he said. "I'm going to work. Linda...what the hell..."

DICs Comparison

Bitter Divorce Guy had serious issues with hyperbole. It should come as no surprise that to a man like him, everything was black or white. While upper management could come up with "the worst ideas in the history of capitalism," he would be able to find solace in a pack of Nutty Bars from the vending machine, "the greatest fucking thing I've ever had in my mouth...ever. End of story."

And don't even get him started on pregnancy. Every time Scott mentioned anything about his wife's progress, Bitter Divorce Guy had a story that was "at least a million times worse." If Scott noticed his wife's boobs were a litter bigger, Bitter Divorce Guy would inevitably weigh in, "Aww, that's nothing. My wife's tits got so big when she was pregnant, I used to accidentally roll on top of them while I was sleeping." If Scott's wife was hungry, Bitter Divorce Guy's wife had her beat: "That's nothing, man. My ex once ate a whole turkey by herself, before Christmas dinner. We had to order fucking pizza. I'm serious. Don't never get married, man." Having learned Bitter Divorce Guy's pattern of one-upmanship, Scott smartly avoided ever mentioning genital odor (good call, Scott).

Another entertaining aspect of Bitter Divorce Guy's communications included his misuse of the word *literally*. We've all used it in the wrong context before to prove a point, but Bitter Divorce Guy made an art form out of its misuse. "My head was going to *literally* explode!" or "She was a big, fat pig...*literally*!" are just a couple. Scott would always chuckle to himself, picturing Bitter Divorce Guy in these peculiarly described situations:

- Describing a bad hangover: "Last night I puked a fucking river...*literally*."
- On his heavy-handed ex-wife: "She *literally* had my balls in a sling."
- After the neighborhood chili cook-off: "I was *literally* crapping my brains out."
- And his unfortunate description of a college one-night stand: "Man, I was banging the shit out of her...*literally*!"

Bitter Divorce Guy always had a knack for making Scott's skin crawl, figuratively speaking, and that's why we loved him.

Myth vs. Fact

Myth: A body pillow can help a pregnant woman's comfort level in bed.
Fact: A body pillow can keep your pregnant wife from rolling over and crushing you to death.

Myth: Women may be offended by The Dudes' description of an enlarged vagina.
Fact: Offending people is easier than taking candy from a retard.

Myth: Intercourse during month eight can induce labor.
Fact: Intercourse during month eight can induce vomiting.

CHAPTER NINE

Weeks 36+

Congratulations. You've come a long way and deserve a pat on the back. It's the beginning of month nine, which means you've reached the halfway point of the pregnancy. "WHAT?!?" you ask, "Wasn't the halfway point about fifteen weeks ago? I mean, you assholes told me that pregnancy lasts forty weeks. I've been reading this fucking book with a pregnant wife sucking the life out of me for the last eight months, looking for a light at the end of the tunnel. I finally reach chapter 9, and you tell me it's halfway over? Is this some kind of sick joke? Why are you laughing? Huh? Do you think this is funny?! Yeah, you guys are really cool. Yuck it up, assholes. Halfway my ass. You guys can seriously go fuck yourselves. Whatever."

Stop foaming at the mouth for a second and listen up. As strange/awful as it may sound, the surprise we've been promising you all along is finally here, and much like the acquisition of herpes, it's one of those unwelcome, burny kinds of surprises: the beginning of month nine is the halfway point of the pregnancy. Ta da! All the crying, aching, nagging, puking, screaming, panting, leaking, scratching, stretching, swelling, and discharging you've experienced for the last eight months is finally at the halfway point (the same is true for your wife's experiences).

Doctors say the baby is at full term during the thirty-seventh week. And now that the proverbial bun in the proverbial oven has finished baking (proverbially speaking), there is nothing to look forward to except for the birth. Eight-plus months of misery are all coming to a head at this point. Your wife wants the baby *out*! And believe us, you will, too. The anticipation causes seconds to seem like minutes, minutes like hours, etc. More precisely, each calendar day from this point will feel like what you remember to be one week. You've just been through 245 calendar days of hell; you now have 35 calendar days, or 245 month-nine days (35 calendar days × 7) to go. This is actually some pretty advanced, abstract mathematical shit. Dr. Stephen Hawking, a close personal friend of our buddy Science, credits the time-warping qualities of month nine of pregnancy as inspiration for his groundbreaking *A Brief History of Time*. If you don't believe us, that's cool.

Similar to the feelings of an African orphan when a rich, white Hollywood couple is in town, all hope is not lost in month nine. In fact, The Dudes recommend you skip the month altogether. "But that's impossible!" you say. Have you no faith in The Dudes after all we've been through? Like that one time we found One-Eyed Willy's treasure with that fat kid and the oddly lovable, retarded, Baby Ruth–eating mutant guy? Or that time we were left alone at home during Christmas and those guys tried to break into our house but we hilariously thwarted the robbery with common household items? We've been through some shit, man, and we're still here for you. In the same spirit, The Dudes, with the help of our friend Science, have equipped this book with time-travel technology. No DeLorean or flux capacitor required. Simply

1. Close *The Dudes' Guide*.
2. Grasp firmly with both hands.
3. Bash book against your head repeatedly until you black out. Have a strong friend continue beating you about the head and torso after you lose consciousness.

(Warning: While in your unconscious state, stay away from the light!)

There. Problem solved. You should come to in time to find out you have a new baby. Unfortunately, you could regain consciousness only to find that you have a ten-year-old son, and your wife has married some rich guy after her unsuccessful bid to get the state to pull your feeding tube (we're still working the bugs out of this time travel thing). In the even more unfortunate event that you come to after just a couple of hours, the rest of chapter 9 will give you an idea of what's in store for you.

Ask The Dudes

Dear Dudes,

With pregnancy only lasting a mere nine months, what keepsakes and mementos (pregnancy test, plaster belly castings, etc.) do you suggest we create to remember the experience forever? I've even heard of couples cooking and eating the placenta. Is this something you recommend?

Sincerely,

Weird D.

Dear Weird,

Outstanding. If you listen closely, you can actually hear the sound of Scott vomiting in the distance.

Oddly enough, you do get a memento to take home from the hospital. It's called "your kid." And unlike some belly pictures that may eventually be hidden away in a photo album, your kid will torture you for the next eighteen to twenty-five years, beginning with two straight years of screaming and pooping. That oughtta help you reminisce about those cherished days of pregnancy.

Sincerely,
The Dudes

In the Bag

As you near the homestretch of your pregnancy adventure, understand that things will get exponentially worse before they get better. In fact, they will probably get exponentially worse and stay there for a while. To help grasp the awfulness of the next few weeks and imminent delivery, we present The Dudes' Douchebag Scale of Douchebaggery™ to help you put particular situations into perspective.

Circumstances presenting no frustration, anger, undue burden, etc., get a "0 bags of douche" rating. An extremely frustrating, anger-inducing, burdensome situation (read: any situation to come) gets a "5 bags of douche" rating, with different levels of douche-baggery in between. Like the Richter scale, it is a logarithmic scale, which basically means that you wouldn't understand if we tried to explain it to you.

To help you get a hang of The Dudes' Douchebag Scale of Douchebaggery™, please complete this short exercise by estimating the appropriate "bags of douche" rating:

1. Your pregnant wife demands a foot rub: _____ bags of douche
2. Your wife goes into labor four weeks early, just as you're about to collect on that "Win a Date with Eva Longoria" contest you won: _____ bags of douche
3. You never got married and thus don't have a pregnant wife: _____ bags of douche

The answers are 1.4, 4.7, and 0 bags of douche, respectively. The Dudes recommend you start utilizing The Dudes' Douchebag Scale of Douchebaggery™ for all life's trappings, pregnancy or otherwise.

Near Myth

Believe us when we say you will reach a point when you are convinced that the baby will never come out, a solid 4+ bags of douche situation (man, that's a lotta douche). And that's when your wife's insane friends and relatives will tell her that inducing labor at home can be fun and easy.

We found the following on an Internet blog:

In private meditation or with someone helping you do guided visualization, go deep within and listen, asking your baby why s/he has not yet decided to go through the birth process. It is the baby who initiates labor. Unlimited answers are possible and might include: fear of the birth process (yours or the baby's); aversion to one or more participants or location planned for the birth; or your feelings of lack of readiness for parenthood. (It may seem as if the answer is coming from your imagination, but your imagination is an important part of your mind.) Then listen for any possible solutions that may be offered.

For those of you who don't have the gift of "the force" or whatever the hell just happened above, here are some other home-inducing methods that are at least as successful:

■ *Castor Oil:* It was the panacea of the Greatest Generation. This elixir of the gods could prevent syphilis, polio, or the plague when combined with vaccinations for syphilis, polio, or the plague. Though considered mostly useless since the age of enlightenment (aka the 1970s), this rotten egg–flavored grease cocktail is still considered a viable labor-inducing agent. Just ask our friend Sean, whose wife drank an entire bottle and went into labor the same day (Sean probably won't mention that she was four days past her due date and that the castor oil also induced a horrific episode of delivery-room diarrhea).

■ *Spicy Foods:* Ever notice how pregnant Cajun and Thai women always go into labor before their due dates? Good, neither have we. Yet the spicy food myth continues to live on. You can have all the jambalaya and curry paste you can eat; just know that this is even less effective than castor oil, which of course is completely ineffective.

■ *Herbal Tea:* We might as well group herbal tea, acupuncture, meditation, and all the other hippie bullcrap together here, as you're probably trying all of them to expedite the impending water birth. Tea technology has come a long way since its heyday. Our parents had three choices: Lipton, iced, or psychedelic. Nowadays, there are teas for just about everything. Tea for falling asleep; tea for waking up. Tea to help you go number one...or number two. Tea to help reduce stress or to make you smarter. We even heard about a tea that can help improve gas mileage, which is just about as believable as a leaf steeped in hot water making your wife's body decide it's time to crap out a kid.

■ *Sex:* Ah yes, the granddaddy of all labor-inducing myths. This is the one that actually works, right? *Right?* "I mean, my wife's friend is a nurse, and she said that semen actually helps thin the cervix, which can kick-start contractions, and nurses are really smart and everything." Your male friends may even give you the heads-up that this one really works, so they've heard. G'head and give it a shot. When you finish climbing down off your wife and she doesn't go into labor and you're left holding your boner and crying, think of The Dudes pointing and laughing at you and taking a video and putting it on YouTube for all the world to see. A recent study determined that semen can actually hinder the onslaught of contractions. It's up to you to take the chance. Pregnancy is going to decide when the baby's coming, and it's not until it's damn well ready. Are we clear? Good.

Drug-Induced Behavior

As the days wear on at an impossibly slow pace, you might think to yourself, "If only there were some kind of magical chemical that doctors could use to jump-start labor!" How forward-thinking of you.

Sometimes a woman's body (hopefully not your woman's body) may not get the idea that forty-two weeks is plenty of time for her uterus to construct a human. In that case, her doctor will schedule a delivery date. On that day, your wife will be injected with a kind of magical chemical that doctors use to jump-start labor, Pitocin. Yeah, it's real. For other medical reasons, like high fetal weight or other pregnancy complications, doctors may schedule a date early on for inducing labor on or around her due date, a refreshing target in the time-warped wormhole that is month nine of pregnancy. This might make you think, "Why the hell don't they do this all the time so's I can get this baby out my wife?" The doctor would say something about "Nature taking its course...blah, blah, blah."

Weeks after you're done losing that argument, and your wife goes into labor naturally five to seven days late, you may notice the nurses hooking her up to a Pitocin drip anyway, just to help move things along. Ha! As has been the case for the last several months and the coming years, the joke is on you. It's your doctor's way of saying, "I could have done this anyway, but I didn't. Worship me now."

☜ Bad Word Choice: The Ripening ☜

If your wife's doctor wants to speed up the delivery,
he or she might do a special procedure called "ripening
the cervix." The doctor will put a special gel all up in there
in order to thin and dilate the cervix. Unfortunately,
the term "ripening" implies edibility, which The Dudes
do not endorse. At all. Ever.

The Grossest Section in This Book

Because this is a book for dudes, and dudes tend to like to gross each other out as much as possible, we thought we'd tell you about a little thing called the mucus plug (shudder).

The mucus plug is, well, a plug made of mucus that covers the opening of your wife's cervix. Think of it as the baby's last line of protection against harmful bacteria and other such foreign nastiness. You'd think Science could have come up with a less horrific name for it, but it seems that he pretty much threw in the towel when it came to the plug.

Aside from the disgusting factor, we decided to tell you about the mucus plug because you might actually hear your wife mention it at some point. We wanted to prepare you (and your gag reflex) for when you hear those words come out of her mouth. A woman's body tends to, uh, eject the plug when it's almost time to give birth. The Dudes liken this ejection to a vaginal sneeze of sorts.

The vaginal sneeze is her body's way of clearing the path. You can think of it as a courtesy to the poor baby, who would otherwise be forced directly through it. Sometimes she'll notice the plug's exit, sometimes she won't. If you're lucky, she'll spare you the sticky details.

Another one of the more disturbing things you might hear during month nine is the term "bloody show." It's a term used to describe the awful mixture of blood and the remnants of the mucus plug that tends to leak from the crotches of pregnant women around the fortieth week. It's a sure bet that if you're hearing the phrase "bloody show" thrown around, the baby will soon be making its miraculous appearance…probably covered in said "show."

The Dudes find it amazing that those two words, when used together, can manage to convey so much imagery. In fact, saying something like "slimy, blood-covered vaginal mucus excretion" is somehow far less offensive to our brains than "bloody show." Please don't ask us why.

Can't, Won't, Mustn't

As you well know by now, pregnancy is constantly fucking with you, no matter what. As your wife is approaching her due date, this mental torture can manifest itself in several unpleasant ways. One of the more annoying annoyances is something Science likes to call false labor. Somehow, your wife's pregnant body can trick itself into thinking the baby is on the way right-the-hell-now, and you need to get in the car and drive dangerously fast to the hospital.

She will experience cramps and contractions exactly like the actual cramps and contractions of actual labor. There will be pain and anguish, and much freaking out the first time it happens. But in the end, all you'll have to show for it are your tortured tears, her shattered dreams, and a half tank of wasted gas.

Unfortunately, there is no real way to know if your wife is actually in labor or not. All you can do is wait it out. If you go to the hospital too early, they might tell you to go right back home. If you don't go to the hospital in time, you run the risk of ruining your sheets and possibly your mattress. As you can see, it's a double-edged sword, and The Dudes advise you to play it as cool as you can. No matter how much she's freaking out, you need to pretend not to be freaking out.

While you're not freaking out, she should be timing the contractions. If they're getting closer together, then go to the hospital. If they're not, still go to the hospital anyway. There is no real reason to risk ruining your perfectly good carpet by misjudging this sort of thing. After all, your wife's erupting vagina is capable of destroying every piece of furniture in the house if you're not careful.

One way that pregnancy lets you know definitively that your little precious bundle of joy is on the way is when her water breaks. "Water breaking" is the term used to describe the event where the bag of fluid surrounding the baby suddenly breaks open and spills out all of its contents right on to your brand-new couch. Scott found this out the hard way, because it was his brand-new couch.

Her water breaking is the equivalent of her body getting pissed that the baby hasn't paid its baby rent in three months and has ignored all the eviction notices. Basically her body just says, "All right, I've had enough, get the hell out!" When this happens, you'll need to get her to the hospital as soon as possible. Well, at least right after you clean off the couch.

Your wife will have likely made up a list of things to bring to the hospital sometime back in month three. This bag has been sitting by the door since then, in anticipation of the big day. In the bag are essentials, like

- makeup: She's gotta look great in those delivery pics.
- a robe: Soon to be covered in uterine goo.
- powder, oils, lotions: For you to massage her with.
- hairbrush: For you to lovingly brush her hair.
- a "going-home outfit" for her: Something loose-fitting yet adorable.

- a "going-home outfit" for the baby: A perfect outfit for the perfect baby.
- a "going-home oufit" for you: Mom doesn't want her new baby to know how much of a slob you actually are.

Now here's a list of what you'll actually need:

- camera, preferably digital: You can show the waiting family pictures of the baby shortly after it's born instead of everyone coming into the room and germing up the place.
- video camera: Note—Use caution to avoid crotch shots so the experience can be enjoyed by (nonperverted) family members at a future date.
- personal video game device, MP3 player, cards, harmonica, small shiny objects: Whatever floats your boat to help pass the time.
- Monsters of Rock CD: A lot of delivery rooms have CD players. Why not bring the kid into a world of rock?
- a backpack full of awesome snacks: Your wife won't be able to eat for a day or so, and the hospital cafeteria only serves, well, hospital food. She may become angry with you for eating in front of her, but would you want your kid brought into a world void of Ho Hos, Doritos, and the like? Quit being so selfish. If you're lucky, they might have a toaster oven so you can heat up some Hot Pockets or something.
- your going-home outfit: No need to pack it; you're already wearing it when you leave the house. However, a clean pair of underwear might not hurt, if you're into that sort of thing.

Note that when the confusion and hysteria of actual contractions begin, you will not be afforded the luxury of five minutes to pack this stuff (even though your baby will probably not be making an appearance until some time tomorrow). And since you are lazy and have failed to pack all this stuff in advance, The Dudes recommend using the thirty seconds you have before departure to grab your wife's prepacked hospital bag, unless you want to miss the birth of your child to run back home and pick it up for your angry wife. Which, come to think of it, may not be such a bad idea...

TV Guide

If television has taught us anything, it's that 90 percent of babies are delivered in cabs. For the 10 percent of you who will actually be delivering in a hospital, the rest of this book should prove very helpful.

Here are some other useful facts that you should have already learned from television:

- Labor, delivery, and recovery is a thirty-minute laugh riot with limited commercial interruptions.
- Pregnant women are witty, charming heroines, while their husbands are bumbling, retarded losers.
- Newborn babies are clean and free of any unpleasant goo.

Furthermore...

- There are angels living amongst us.
- The disabled can teach us all a valuable lesson.

- Hot babes always marry fat, hilarious men.
- Your wacky neighbor will annoy you, save your life, or eventually teach you the meaning of true love.

It's TV, people. It has no reason to lie to you, and neither do we.

Myth vs. Fact

Myth: Your baby's due date will be here before you know it.
Fact: It's kind of mean to even joke about that.

Myth: You can communicate with your baby through meditation.
Fact: Meditation is as effective a baby communication tool as yelling into your wife's vagina.

Myth: Labor pains are your baby's way of lovingly saying, "I'm ready to meet you."
Fact: Your wife's screams of pain are her way of lovingly saying, "Get me to the fucking hospital now!"

CHAPTER TEN

Labor, Delivery, and Recovery

It's two days past the due date, your wife is doubled over in pain, and your dog is sniffing around the puddle of amniotic fluid on the living room floor. Eureka! Sounds like it's time to have a baby. Load up the car, grab your wife, and call the vet to have the dog put down. You won't be needing him anymore.

Delivery Driver

The Dudes can say with absolute certainty that when you are driving your wife to the hospital, you will encounter one or more of the following:

- heavy snow and/or ice storm
- road construction and major detours onto roads you've never seen
- old lady driving 7 to 10 miles per hour under the posted speed limit
- mud slide and/or flock of sheep in the middle of the road
- getting carjacked

- you feeling hungry and actually contemplating stopping for fast food
- you actually stopping for fast food
- you wishing you hadn't stopped for fast food

Support Groupie

If you want your entire family in the delivery room looking at your wife's crotch giving birth, that's fine, but The Dudes think that a phone call allowing them to arrive in the waiting room just in time to see the baby get wheeled into the nursery would be just as good. We could say more, but if you really want to put that into perspective, just imagine you and her mother standing there looking at your wife's crotch while the doctor is shouting out commands. Not exactly an ideal situation, because even if it's not spoken, your mother-in-law will, as usual, be totally blaming you for all of her daughter's pain.

The Dudes will assume that by the time that you're driving to the hospital, you and your wife will have already decided exactly who will be watching your child emerge triumphantly. In light of that, the drive to the hospital will be the perfect time to call these so-called delivery-room VIPs so they can be there with plenty of time to witness the miracle.

Once you get to the hospital, you'll need to grab all the stuff that you brought with you and hurry inside. Usually you'll go through the emergency room entrance. This is great, because it gives you a chance to get directly to the head of the line while everyone else sits around in the waiting room, trying to keep themselves from bleeding all over the six-month-old copy of *Newsweek* they're struggling to read through the pain.

Once past the emergency room lobby, you'll quickly be checked in, your wife will be put in a wheelchair, and you'll both be whisked off to the maternity ward. Well, she'll be whisked. You'll be trailing behind, carrying all the bags full of crap she heard she'd need at the hospital.

Every Body Hurts

One of the first things the nurse will tell your wife about as she settles in is the hospital pain scale. She will be asked to rate her level of pain, from 1 to 10, where 1 is the equivalent of the pain of a haircut, 9 is the pain of delivering a baby, and 10 is the pain of a Brazilian bikini wax. She may even give your wife a handy chart with a series of smiley to scowly faces to help her get an idea of how to translate her feelings into numbers. Of course, the frowny face (with tears) that represents the number 10 is a polite understatement. Depending on how expressive your wife can be, you and the entire floor of the hospital may be in for a real show. Profanity-laced tirades are not uncommon. The best thing you can do is to hope for a quick finish while trying hard to pretend that you don't think your wife is out of her fucking mind.

To give you a better idea of how much pain your wife is in, The Dudes have prepared The Dudes' Guide to Pain, below.

	Wife	Dude
☺	1	Mild buffalo wings
	2	Swallowing a tortilla chip without having chewed it enough
	3	Medium buffalo wings

	Wife	Dude
	4	Getting your girlfriend's initials tattooed on your shoulder
☺	5	Watching *The View*
	6	Getting your ex-girlfriend's initials lasered off your shoulder
	7	Realizing your dad was always too busy for you (Cat's in the cradle, man)
	8	Tweezing a nosehair
	9	Tweezing a nosehair (the skinny ones on the nostril divider side)
☹	10	Crapping a 7- to 10-pound, 19-inch turd (a day after eating a dozen "Fire" buffalo wings)

As an added bonus, The Dudes' Pain Scale has an advanced level of pain we refer to as Level 11. This level can only be experienced if you let your wife see the above Dudes' Guide to Pain.

Screw This

As soon as your wife gets settled in, the nurse will fire up the equipment for monitoring the baby. The baby can be monitored externally or internally. The external monitor is basically a strap that stretches around the belly with some sort of electronic sensor on it. The sensor monitors the baby's heartbeat and the ferocity of the contractions. The sensor is attached to a computer that has some sort of seismic-looking graph paper coming out of it. There is also a screen that allows your wife to see just how horrible the next contraction is going to be a couple of seconds before it actually happens.

The sensor strap is specifically designed to be uncomfortable and to slip off at random times. Those random times are usually the exact times that you'll be watching the heartbeat on the monitor. Seeing your baby's heart rate drop to zero is guaranteed to seriously freak you the fuck out and cause you to start flailing with the button that calls the nurses in—nurses who will nonchalantly walk in, adjust the strap, look at you like you're retarded, and leave.

If the doctor or nurses decide that direct monitoring is necessary, they'll use the external strap, plus the internal monitors. The internal monitors can only be used if the bag is broken and there is some dilation. The internal contraction monitor isn't really that bad. All the nurse does is put some sort of lubed-up, fluid-filled tube (heh) between the baby and the wall of the uterus.

The internal baby heart rate monitor is a small hook screw that is lovingly jabbed into your baby's scalp and left there throughout the rest of the labor. If you've blocked the reality of an implement of construction being fastened to your unborn child's scalp, all you'll see is the nurse fiddling with another cord between your wife's legs, and that will be that. Soon you'll be enjoying the show on a monitor as the baby's heart-rate pattern appears. So as you're watching the heart rate on the monitor, try to forget that it's coming from the screw in your baby's head, which is still inside your wife. If Science was conscious, we'd give him the thumbs-up sign on this one for sure. Now, if at some point in the future you notice your child isn't the genius you thought he'd be, simply blame it on the head screw. If nobody buys into that, then blame it on your wife's bad genes. That's what The Dudes plan on doing.

Labor Day Marathon

Had you been paying attention in baby class all those
weeks ago, you probably wouldn't have learned a goddamn
thing about how this labor process works anyway. So it
turns out that it was quite forward-thinking of you to day-
dream about defeating Ed "Cookie" Jarvis in the Annual
Buffalo Wing–Eating Competition (short form) during all
those hours of useless instruction. To catch you up, here is
a summary of how things work, in three easy steps.

1. Over a period of several hours (usually), the contractions of labor cause your wife's cervix (wombhole) to dilate (widen).
2. Contractions also cause the cervical tissue to thin,
   or efface.
3. When the cervix has dilated 10 centimeters and
   effaced 100 percent (when the wombhole is really
   wide and thin), she begins actively pushing (aka
   bearing down, thrusting, making a poopinglike
   motion) with the onset of each contraction to forcibly remove the large baby via her formerly snug
   birth canal.

That is how the process works; forget about ridiculous
egghead, doctory terms that nobody understands, such as
station 3, crowning, or *baby.* This is all you need to know.

How the doctor checks for dilation and effacement is
surprisingly low-tech. Imagine a woman coming into the
room once an hour, putting on a glove, and shoving her
entire hand up your wife's crotch...usually minus any
warning or polite conversation. Then imagine you being

genuinely curious about how many centimeters she's dilated and to what percent she is effaced, and perhaps wanting to check for yourself (for curiosity's sake). These two numbers are what control your destiny, for the next few hours anyway. And you will look forward to the nurse's hourly crotch hand exam with extreme anticipation.

Bill's wife's dilation and effacement moved along pretty slowly. The nurses cranked up the speed of her Pitocin drip every hour or so until she was a full-on birthing machine. God bless synthetic hormones and the brave animals used to make them.

Tip from the Front Lines

If the labor is progressing slowly, your wife might allow some visitors to come in and hang out. Be prepared, though, because some of them might think they can stay for the whole event. Feel free to encourage Uncle Steve to get the fuck out by using open-handed slaps and forearms to the face and neck. As an added bonus, witnessing this tends to clear the room of any other lingering friends or relatives as well.

Watershed Moment

What's a nine-month pregnancy adventure that doesn't end with a splashtastic river of amniotic fluid? If your wife's bag of waters hasn't ruined your couch already and is still intact at the hospital, her crotch could be in for a raging-river safari-venture. You see, as her uterine contractions get stronger and stronger, they squeeze the sac and fluids within, like a water balloon ready to burst. This can culminate in an explosive result. And if any medical professional is in position, we suggest you be ready with the video camera.

Usually, before it gets to that point, the doctor will break the bag with a plastic crochet hook. We're sure it has some sort of technical name, but it is basically a plastic crochet hook that the doctor inserts into the cervix to tear an opening in the lining, releasing its contents. Note this plastic crochet hook will cost you or your insurance company $25 to $50.

Additionally, the doctor's breaking the bag of waters may not bring on the highly anticipated, raging torrent of fluid. This is a result of the baby's head blocking the opening of the cervix. In this scenario, you've got a ticking time bomb delivery. There's fluid in there, and it's coming out eventually. If you ever played Perfection as a kid, racing against the ticking clock to put every tiny, shaped piece in its proper position before the entire game exploded in your face, you're ready for this. When the baby's head gets through, somebody's gonna get it. And you can rest assured it will be hilarious, especially if it's not you.

There's a chance the amniotic fluid may have a greenish hue to it. If so, that simply means the fetus has released meconium into the uterus. Translation: Congrats! Your son/daughter has taken his/her first crap. In this scenario, the doctor will want to make sure the birth process moves along because of the possibility that the baby may have ingested some meconium (ew), which could cause problems beyond you just being grossed out.

Nurse-Doctor Relationship

We know that when you're in the hospital, you'll be unnecessarily worried about a whole bunch of crap that you'll have absolutely no control over. That's why we'd like to point out a fun little bit of hospital drama that you might have missed had you not had the good fortune of reading this book. It's something we like to call The Doctor-Nurse Dynamic.

Doctors and nurses have a strange relationship. Nurses tend to look at doctors as bumbling, overpaid fools with no common sense. They seem to look at themselves as underpaid, unappreciated workhorses. Modern-day heroes, if you will. We can imagine the nurses all sitting around the bar after a hard day of saving lives, saying, "Yeah, well, those f'ing doctors might be book smart, but that's all they've got. We've got the street smarts, and that's what really matters."

Actually, The Dudes think what really matters is the huge paychecks the doctors go home with, but you won't catch us trying to tell that to a bunch of pissed-off, drunken nurses who are undoubtedly looking for a fistfight.

A perfect example of this Doctor-Nurse Dynamic occurred when Scott's wife asked him to take a picture of her and her doctor. Unfortunately, the bed rail was blocking part of the shot. The doctor looked at the bed rail, then at the nurse, then back at the bed rail. The nurse gave her the "Well, genius? What the hell are you waiting for?" look. The doctor had no clue whatsoever how to move the rail. She fumbled with it for about fifteen awkward seconds before she gave up and asked the nurse to help her. The nurse gave an exasperated sigh that screamed, "You're the goddamn doctor! You figure it out!" She rolled her eyes so far back that it hurt Scott to even watch. She stomped over to the bed and pushed a small red button for the doctor, and the offending rail went down with ease. Scott quickly took the picture before any more awkward doctor-nurse moments could break out.

Scott felt pretty confident that the nurse would later be sarcastically pantomiming the doctor's lame attempts to adjust the bed rail in the nurses' break room. Saying to all the other nurses, "Seriously though, the doctor didn't even know how to adjust the bed rail...and she makes how much?" At which point they'd all nod knowingly and acknowledge similar experiences with those retarded, overpaid doctors.

Uncomfortably Numb

Some women view labor pain control as a direct challenge to their womanhood. They don't say this explicitly, though. They usually disguise their feelings by saying that they are concerned about how the pain meds might affect the baby. The Dudes wholeheartedly call bullshit on this, though. We call bullshit because any woman who has gone through pregnancy without pain meds will, without hesitation, use that fact as a condescending trump card in any discussion about pain.

It doesn't matter if you've had massive head trauma, lost a limb, or had kidney stones, these women have you beat every single time. They even tend to annoy the shit out of women who chose the pain meds. Women love to tell their pregnancy "battle stories" whenever the subject comes up, and the pain med–free women always make a point of mentioning, and rementioning, how awesome they are for caring so much about their babies. The proverbial dead horse is beaten into a meaty pulp with just a few condescending sentences. If your wife is sensitive to this, you might have to deal with her second-guessing her decision to get the pain meds.

Science tells us that modern pain medication, if used properly during pregnancy, will have little or no effect on the baby, especially the epidural. Now, go ask a midwife, and she'll have a completely different view on the subject. The Dudes always side with Science on matters such as these. We were there when Science used to date a midwife. They argued constantly, and he would always complain about how she would only take his side when it was convenient. He even suspected her of secretly stealing money out of his wallet. The breakup was not pretty.

There are various anesthetics available for laboring women. Your doctor will help decide what medication, if any, is the best choice for your wife. The timing of delivering the pain medication is crucial because it can affect how your wife will push when the time arrives.

If the pain medication is administered too heavily or at the wrong time, then no amount of you calling your wife a wuss and telling her she's "gotta want it more" will get her to push. This will result in everyone having to wait until feeling returns. Remember, as any doctor might tell you, the goal is to get this over with as soon as possible. Oh, and a happy, healthy baby, too.

One of the greatest gifts Science has bestowed upon women is the epidural. With an epidural, an anesthesiologist will insert a small tube into your wife's lower back. A tiny slice of heaven will flow through this tube into the sac of fluid surrounding the spinal cord. We're not really sure what happens beyond that, but we can definitely say that it tends to make everything better. There is little to no danger to the baby with the epidural. Pretty much the worst that can happen is a severe headache or it doesn't work at all, but that's rare.

Sometimes, with an epidural, your wife will be given a button that allows her to dose herself if she's feeling pain. Self-administered pain medication—it's about time Science caught up. Housewives in the suburbs have been doing that for years.

Numbing Agent

Women always tell the same story about their anesthesiologist. It usually goes something like this: "And when he walked in the room, I immediately fell in love with him," or "After he inserted my epidural, I asked him to marry me. Seriously, I did. I'm not joking, girls, I actually said that. Isn't that crazy? I know!" The truth is, it'll be a cold day in hell when a wealthy doctor takes one look at a bloated, sweaty, moaning woman in labor and says to himself, "Once I get this needle inserted, I have to work up the nerve to ask this lady out."

It turns out that the doctor-nurse relationship that we spoke of earlier applies to anesthesiologists, too. To hear Scott's wife talk about her anesthesiologist is to hear her describe an angelic figure, complete with halo, who enters the room in a puff of white smoke and brilliant white light. To hear Scott describe it, the guy was tall and middle-aged, and had a serious comb-over issue.

After his wife stopped thanking the anesthesiologist and telling him how awesome he was, she told him to fly back to heaven as he was leaving. Hearing this, the irritated nurse muttered something sarcastic about him not hitting his stupid halo on the way out and to please get the hell out of her way.

Helpful Advice

There really isn't anything you can do to reduce your wife's discomfort during delivery. If you try rubbing a cold towel on her forehead, you might just end up pissing her off more. So good luck with that.

Push It Real Good

When the baby has descended far enough into the birth canal, and your wife's cervix (wombhole) has dilated a full 10 centimeters, it's time for the real deal: pushing. This is when your wife goes into full-on, active, physical labor.

Despite what you learn from television, your function in the delivery room is basically nothing. You've been fetching ice chips for your wife for several hours, and you're about to get knocked down a few notches in responsibility and pay grade. Breathing exercises, counting, positioning—all that stuff goes out the window when the moment comes to start pushing. The nurse(s) will usually take over and lead your wife through the ordeal. From time to time she might have you push the epidural button that gives her a dose of medication, but that's basically it. But there is no need to feel bad or left out. Just remember all that hard work you did nine months ago. You've definitely paid your dues.

Now, when one of her monster contractions begins, which is about every minute at this point, she starts to push the baby out. You've experienced this sensation usually the day after rib/chili/beerfest, only there isn't a group of medical professionals surrounding you to talk you through your "delivery." Anyway, your wife will push during these contractions while you and the nurses count to ten, taking a breath after the ten count and repeating two more times for each contraction, or some such. That's it. Pretty easy, huh? Sure. But just like the last nine months, pregnancy still has a few tricks up its sleeve.

The first of these is the duration of this delivery phase. Bill's wife pushed three times a minute for three f'ing hours of his daughter's delivery. At one point, Bill became so tired of counting to ten, he had to take a break, knowing the nurses would cover for him. This did not go over as well as Bill thought it would, so he grudgingly rejoined the grunting infant-dispensing before him. Ironically, his wife quickly grew annoyed with the sound of his voice and yelled at him to "stop fucking counting now!" So he was forced to lovingly head-bob along with the announcement of each integer.

The second delivery scamola, and we suspect this is a big one, is the nurses' conspiracy to make you and your wife think that the baby is seconds away from arrival. Surprisingly early during the active labor/pushing phase, you'll be able to see the top of your baby's head. Bill remembers this as a significant moment, thinking to himself, "So this whole thing wasn't just all bullshit. There really is a baby in there, and I'm really excited to see what she looks like." In a precursor to your child's adolescent years, however, he or she will repeatedly and disrespectfully recede back up the birth canal between contractions in stubborn, turdlike fashion. If your baby's delivery is like most women's first births, you can expect this to go on for a while. Or can you?

The nurses will excitedly tell your wife, "Wow, the baby's almost here!" perhaps sounding a bit surprised at the baby's rapid progress. Another contraction, big push, "I can see the head." So can you. "Keep pushing," they say. Again, there's the head. This is so exciting. It's almost over!

A dad-to-be of above-average intelligence should be able to pick up anywhere from fifteen to ninety minutes into this bullshit that the baby is hardly going anywhere. Your epiphany will only cause further confusion. The nurses are obviously doing this to keep your sucker of a wife motivated. She's exhausted, in a lot of pain, and she's apparently got a long way to go. You'll be confused about whether you should side with the nurses (con artists) or your wife (the mark). The correct answer is the nurses in the short run and your wife in the long run. Of course, you can always deny everything and just say you were agreeing with the experienced medical professionals. Good luck.

Tip from the Front Lines

Think long and hard about whether or not you want to watch the actual delivery of your child. Up until recently, the vagina was your personal, happy fun land. If you don't want that imagery threatened, you might consider bringing a welding mask. Remember, there are things in life that you simply can't un-see. Your child being forced out of your wife's vagina is one of them.

Toolbox

Charles Darwin's observations among certain animal groups helped him formulate a basis for his *On the Origin of Species*. The Dudes tend not to take sides in the whole creationism versus evolutionism argument, but we would like to note that had Darwin decided to spend more time studying Beaver Valley than the Galápagos Islands, scientific history may have taken a drastically different course.

Sure, natural selection ensures survival of the species, and genetic mutations are great, and we all used to have pouches and whatnot, but if ol' Chuck is right, the vagina must have opted out of the entire evolutionary process. Women have been crapping out kids for millions of years, right? Why, then, are women crapping out 6- to 12-pound babies through a too-small skin tube while pushing and screaming for hours until their vaginas eventually tear open to let the kid out? C'mon, evolution! Shouldn't we be at the point 4 million years into the game where the baby just kinda rolls on out, yanks out the placenta behind it, and makes a beeline for mom's teat? Maybe this is what God has been trying to tell us all along. Too bad He decided to stop talking to people a couple thousand years ago. Maybe it's because instead of spending all His time talking to us lame humans, He was busy inventing forceps.

Forceps are one of the devices used to force your baby from the friendly confines of the womb. If he's not cooperating, these Civil War–era, stainless steel salad tong–like devices grab your baby's head in the birth canal and yanks him into this cruel world, where he will quickly be introduced to the wonders of manhandling nurses and hypodermic needles. Better yet, why not utilize newfangled, early-20th-century technology to free your stubborn, large-headed baby from your wife's innards? Why not attach a vacuum to your baby's head and suck, suck, suck him out? You'll be happy to know there isn't a doctor who can think of a good reason not to.

What's that, you say? Your wife has been pushing for three straight hours and the baby just doesn't want to come out? Well, why not cut open your wife's stomach and yank him out? You know, like Caesar! Again, the doctors will be happy to oblige.

Sarcasm aside (momentarily), the Caesarian (C)-section birth is pretty much the Cadillac of births. There's no screaming, crying, sweating, pushing, getting yelled at— all the wonders of a vaginal birth. It's a rather rudimentary medical idea that makes a lot of sense. Cut open the belly; get the baby. In fact, it really makes that whole vaginal birth thing sound archaic and comically nonsensical, like organized labor. Ignore the fact that it's major abdominal surgery, complete with painful recovery. Plus, it has the added benefit of making granola-eating midwives cry.

Doctors recommend C-section births for breech (legs first) deliveries, high potential birth weight babies, and other delivery complications. The Dudes are all for happy, healthy babies and mothers but, for argument's sake, we would like to present the pros and cons of vaginal birth versus C-section delivery.

Vaginal	C-Section
Long, painful birth	Permanent abdominal scar
Tearing of the perineum (taint)	Scar
Long postdelivery healing	That scar
Wider, looser during future intercourse	Seeing that scar during intercourse

Hail to the Chief (Resident)

During the hours of pushing, the doctor will occasionally grace you with his presence. If he happens to be on a break from hanging doctor certificates on his office wall or counting his gold coins, he'll pop in and check on the baby's progress. As quickly as he comes, he will be gone, as he's probably between holes in a celebrity pro-am golf tournament. When the baby has reached the point where you think, "There's no way the baby's head is going to fit though there," it's time for the doctor to make his final appearance and show you how unfortunately correct you are.

First, he'll order one of the underappreciated, overworked nurses to put his golf clubs in the corner. Then he'll scrub up and get ready to take part in the entire last five minutes of the delivery.

At this crucial point, it's time for the doctor to perform an episiotomy. This is where he basically grabs a sharp pair of scissors and cuts your wife's taint, allowing the baby the room it needs to get the hell outta there. This crude-sounding technique beats the alternative of Nature's episiotomy, technically referred to as tearing. The viewing of the delivery at this point is best left to medical professionals, who are highly trained to view gore for a living.

Forty years ago, you would have been sitting in the hospital waiting room, poised to light up cigars to celebrate the arrival of your new son or daughter. You wouldn't have known of the crying, screaming, cutting, tearing, and other wonders going on in the delivery room. You also wouldn't have known that the cigar you were about to smoke was going to instantly give everybody in the room lung cancer, you insensitive prick.

The thing is, the great, horrific miracle of childbirth is now happening before your eyes, and it's something you've probably already seen on TV somewhere. What was once a mystery to men the world over is now a weekend marathon on the Health Channel. Still, what is happening before your eyes in the delivery room is intensely personal and incredibly difficult to put into words, as The Dudes have issues with emotional sincerity. Suffice it to say, it involves a very grayish-blue baby, an exhausted but triumphant wife, and probably you crying.

Ahem…uh…we mean, that is if you're a complete wuss.

Anecdote from Bill's Uncle Don

"She had been pushing for a few hours, when finally after one big push my son's head emerged into the world. A fascinating thing about birth is that once the head is out, a woman's pelvic muscles contract around the baby's shoulders and abdomen, helping to squeeze all the crap out of his lungs and throat. Well, my wife must have gotten in a good squeeze, because my partially born son started to scream his head off. There he/she/they were, my wife spread-eagled on the delivery table with a screaming, red baby head between her legs. I came to several minutes later to find that my son's head had in fact been born with an entire body attached…whew! Though I will always retain a fond memory of my crotch-headed wife-baby."

Neonatal AV Club

One of the few responsibilities you'll actually have in the delivery room is that of media expert. Most couples head to the hospital with a video recorder and a digital camera so as not to miss a single second of the miracle. You'll be no different.

Scott's wife was a little overzealous about preserving the magic, though. So much so, in fact, that she was taking pictures and video on the drive *to* the hospital. She continued doing this all the way up to the delivery room. His wife reluctantly gave up her video camera and two still cameras when the labor really kicked in.

As she was lying on the bed, going through full-on contractions, she was drilling Scott on what shots and angles she wanted when the baby was delivered. Scott tried his best to pay attention. Unfortunately, he got distracted while thinking about how cool it would be if that light in the ceiling was actually a giant robot arm that could shoot deadly lasers at his enemies.

Looking like a foreign tourist with three different cameras around his neck, Scott got to work. He wandered from place to place around the room, trying to line up the best shots. Immediately after the baby was born, his wife informed him that he was doing a crappy job with the pictures. She accused him of not listening to a word she said and demoted him to photographer's assistant.

That's right, less than ten minutes after giving birth, Scott's wife was directing a full-on photo shoot right from her bed. While preserving the memories is important, one can't overlook the importance of robot arms that shoot lasers, either.

Look, a Head!

In our continuing effort to ensure that you're not completely freaked-the-fuck-out in the delivery room, we feel it necessary to describe exactly why your baby might look like—a creepy, pear-headed alien lab experiment gone wrong.

One of the cruelest tricks that Nature will play on your wife (and ultimately you) is the old "head is bigger than the vagina" trick. Believe us, the only one laughing here is Nature. Well, possibly Science, too, because he's a sadistic asshole sometimes. Anyway, in making the baby's head far bigger than the opening it's supposed to fit through, Nature created somewhat of a problem: how the hell is the baby supposed to get out?

Nature ended up solving this problem by making your baby's skull out of tiny little disconnected plates. As your wife is pushing the baby's head up against the too-small opening, the plates slide over the top of each other. This allows the head (and brain) to be smashed down to whatever size is necessary for it to be shoved mercilessly out into the cold, unforgiving world.

We will concede that this painful-looking baby squeeze does seem to serve a purpose. In compressing the skull and chest, a great deal of the prenatal goo gets squeezed out of the baby's lungs and orifices. Plus, it helps to kick off the whole "breathe or die" cycle, which seems pretty important.

The "best" part about all this is the fact that it's possible that your baby's head might be horribly misshapen for a while. We're talking several inches of skull bulge that'll make you seriously reconsider getting that paternity test. There's no way in hell your baby's head could look that fucked up, right?

Luckily, the hospital will slap on a cute little baby hat right over the skull bulge. They'll say it's for warmth, but you'll know the truth. The bulge-covering hat will allow for cute pictures and barely make you forget about the misshapen head issue. Don't worry, though. Given a couple of weeks, your baby's skull will start to look fairly normal.

The only remaining remnant will be a quarter-sized squishy brain hole on the top of his/her head where the skull plates haven't quite grown together yet. The Dudes like to call this the Brain Window. We know it might be tempting to push on the squishy brain window to see if you can make your baby's legs kick or something, but try to resist the urge if you can.

After Birth

With one final push, your scary-as-hell–looking child has emerged. He/she is wrinkly, pissed off, and has the aforementioned head-shape issues. He/she is also covered with blood and goo, or vernix, an in utero wet suit of sorts. The baby is often tossed up on the mother's chest for a quick, inconvenient (as far as the doctors are concerned) look at mom and then hauled off for a good cleaning and general molestation.

Dad and any other delivery-room VIPs are invited to follow the now pink, screaming infant over to the baby warming tray (to keep the baby fresh) for continued photo and/or video documentation. Here the nurse violently cleans, footprints, wraps, and squirts salve into the eyes of your precious son/daughter. Note that this is not done in a pleasant, gentle fashion, but in a much more mechanical, get-this-over-with style that you'd be familiar with if you worked at a chicken slaughterhouse.

While the oohing and ahhing continues over the new baby, you probably won't notice the continued hell your wife is experiencing across the room. Since you won't be noticing, here's what's happening.

The doctor will ask her for one more good push to deliver the placenta (meat pocket) from the womb. He then begins to stitch what is left of your wife's privates back together. If you're lucky, he's had frontline combat experience in a close-range shotgun battle and can figure out what is supposed to go where. Ogling the baby is Nature's way of having you avoid the horrors of your wife's nether regions. If you happen to think of her, The Dudes recommend that whether out of fear or love, you keep your eyes on the baby for now.

Dr. Dude Says

"When the nurses get your baby all cleaned off, you might notice something alarming. Many babies tend to have a fine coat of dark fur covering portions of their bodies. Yes, I did just say baby fur. Rest assured that your wife probably didn't have sex with a werewolf, and yes, the baby is actually yours. The technical term for this hair is *lanugo* (from the Latin for *'sex with a werewolf'*), and it's perfectly harmless. Lanugo grows on infants as a way of insulating them in the womb. This hair pretty much goes away by the end of the first week, so put away the tweezers."

Dis-cord

Imagine those giant novelty scissors that they use for grand openings at supermarkets. Now imagine the grand opening being your child's delivery, and you're the distinguished guest of honor with the scissors. Don't cut just yet, because in the interest of full disclosure, there are a few things The Dudes need to, uh, disclose.

Cutting the cord isn't quite as straightforward as you might think. Well…the actual cutting is pretty straight-forward, but the issues surrounding it aren't. Some doctors encourage it, some you'll have to get clearance from, and others do it before you even realize your wife has given birth at all. It's best to let the doctor know beforehand if you actually want to cut the cord or if you'd rather have him do it.

Now, if you actually want to hear a board-certified physician call you a douche bag, try bringing in your own cord-cutting instrument. Some guys think it's important to cut the cord with the family heirloom Viking sword or the sentimental pocketknife that their father, and his father before him, used. After calling you a douche bag, the doctor will explain to you about bacteria and sterile hospital environments and infection and a bunch of other horrible stuff—the same stuff that Science already tried to explain to you the last time you two got piss drunk together.

Again, don't cut that cord quite yet, because The Dudes haven't finished freaking you out.

There are some groups of people who consider cutting the cord one of the most traumatic events a child can go through. This is the literal severing of the mother/child bond and can cause great stress, especially if done by the father. The ramifications of the cord cutting might not surface until the kid is thirteen and subconsciously blaming *you* for all the trauma in his/her life. At least if it's the doctor that did the cutting, he can take the heat.

Of course, The Dudes don't subscribe to this ridiculous nonsense any more than we subscribe to the notion that you can find a thirteen-year-old who doesn't think his/her parents are responsible for everything that goes wrong in his/her (far easier than we had it) life.

If you do decide to cut the cord yourself, please note that it's really not all that remarkable in practice. The doctors put two little clamps on it and hand you the sterile scissors. They show you exactly where to cut and let you go to work. Cutting the cord feels a bit like cutting a small piece of rubber. The Dudes weren't really all that excited by the whole deal. It certainly isn't the magical experience you might have been tricked into thinking it was by some of your wife's pregnancy books. This, we might add, is another reason we pretty much only read the chapters about sex.

ⓘ   **Not So Fun Fact**   ⓘ

A lotus birth is a technique wherein the cord and placenta are left attached to the baby after the delivery and are allowed to fall off naturally, usually after a couple weeks. If you've already brought your baby home sans cord and placenta, you can still duplicate the fun of a lotus birth with some flexible hose and a boneless chuck roast.

DICs: Final Cut

At work one day, Scott leaned over the cubicle wall and said to Foreign Guy, "Hey, if you ever have a kid, do you think you'll want to cut the cord yourself, or let the doctor do it?"

He thought about the question for slightly too long, then started to answer. "You see, Scott, in my country, the gods often demand a—"

Just then, Bitter Divorce Guy leaned over his cube wall, interrupting, "This guy doesn't even know what a real girl looks like. I don't see why you're asking him. When my kid was born, I told the doctor to go fuck himself when he asked me if I wanted to cut the cord. I ain't goin' near any of that crap. No way. You couldn't pay me enough. Don't never get married, dude, it ain't worth it. End of story."

Angry about being interrupted, Foreign Guy said something about his gods, a sacrifice, and Bitter Divorce Guy. As they were arguing and cursing, Sensitive Guy leaned over his cube wall and offered Scott some other advice.

"Cutting the cord is tantamount to the psychological torture of an infant, Scott." Knowing that it was best to just let him finish, Scott simply nodded knowingly as Sensitive Guy continued. "When my daughter was born, my wife and I were horrified to see the doctor swiftly and brutally sever our baby from her mother. It was so difficult and traumatic for me, my wife, and the baby. We thought that she would never forgive us."

As Sensitive Guy went on, Scott noticed Foreign Guy cursing Bitter Divorce Guy—not swearing, mind you, but actually putting a curse on him. Sensitive Guy ignored them both: "You see though, Scott, we soon realized that one bond was forcefully taken from my daughter, but a more amazing bond of pure love was about to be created."

Finally, Bitter Divorce Guy jumped in for the rescue. "Dude, look at yourself!" he said to Sensitive Guy. "What the hell is wrong with you? You're actually crying right now!" Realizing that tears were starting to stream down his face, Sensitive Guy gave a loud sob and walked briskly to the bathroom to cry it out in private.

Still undecided about cutting the cord, Scott sat and listened as Foreign Guy finished his hex on Bitter Divorce Guy with some barely audible mumbling, followed by a burning smell.

Two weeks later, after returning from his vacation in the Philippines, a jubilant Bitter Divorce Guy was showing off his new ring, wedding photos, and a surprisingly uncharacteristic outlook on marriage. He and the new love of his life, Lapulapu, were happily celebrating their one-week anniversary. In a shocking turn of events, Bitter Divorce Guy had transformed into Sensitive Divorced Foreign Married Guy.

It turns out Foreign Guy's marriage curse had backfired, and the new Sensitive Divorced Foreign Married Guy ain't never been happier...literally. End of story.

Dr. Dude Says

"Don't freak out if your baby has acne like you did as a teenager. It's caused by maternal hormones mixing with the baby's bloodstream and is entirely your wife's fault. So dry those tears of teenage nostalgia and put away the medicated pads, because there isn't a damn thing you can do about it."

Congratulations, It's a...Whoa!

Your wife has successfully crapped out a kid. Specifically, you're wife has crapped out a boy...a blue baby boy (were it a girl, it would have been pink, of course).

After the initial awe ("Wow, so this is what it's like for me to have a baby") and concern ("Why are they being so rough with this baby who is rumored to be my son?"), you'll start to notice other details. Maybe he has a full head of black hair, your wife's nose, or crablike claws instead of hands (it happens). Incredibly, he will have the scrotum of a 7-foot-tall, 380-pound man. You will likely be as proud as you are confused.

A newborn baby boy's sack is a wonder of nature. Science told us it has something to do with fluid collecting in the scrotum prior to birth, but then he said that he was collecting fluid for our moms and then laughed and walked away. Nonetheless, it's a sight to see and nearly impossible to avoid. You may even feel compelled to nudge others when they see the boy during a diaper change and give them a nodding, "Eh? EH?" Note that it's best to resist this urge and to keep to yourself your pride over the fact that your boy's nutsack is as big as your own.

Exit Interview

Shortly after your baby is born, he will be given his first-ever standardized test. The test is called the Apgar test. It's actually a series of professional observations about your baby's appearance and behavior that will determine whether or not special infant medical procedures are needed, and how many babes he'll eventually score with.

Apgar is the name of the anesthesiologist who created the test, but it is also a useful mnemonic for the observations made: appearance, pulse, grimace, activity, and respiration. The nurse or doctor will observe or test each of these areas and assign a score based on how awesome your baby is. A high score will warrant bragging rights at work. A low score indicates a punch to the face of both you and your insurance company.

The Apgar scoring scale is 0 to 2, with a 2 being normal. Since there are five categories, Science tells us that we're looking for a score of 10. Here's how it all works...

Appearance is basically an observation of skin color. Once all the birthin' remnants have been hosed off, the doctor will check to see if your baby looks blue. Science tells us that the blue color has something to do with the lack of oxygen. Thus, nonblue babies earn a full 2 points.

Pulse is just that—a measure of your baby's heart rate. A pulse of over one hundred beats per minute will score you a 2. Less than that will mean that you have failed as a father.

Grimace, also called reflex irritability, is basically the measurement of your baby saying, "Stop fucking poking me, you asshole!" So if your baby gets pissed at being "stimulated," chalk up another 2 points.

Activity, also called muscle tone, is a measurement of how much your baby is flexing his muscles. It's simply an observation of how much your baby is squirming around right after birth. If you're baby's doing calisthenics, give yourself a 2. If not, hide your head in shame, because he's obviously a total loser who'll never be making the varsity team, ever.

Respiration is exactly that. Is your kid breathing, or is it time to completely freak the fuck out? This one's pretty important, so let's shoot for a 2 and try not to think about the alternative.

After the grading is done, the nurse will write the score somewhere on the baby's chart. A score of 10 will mean that your baby is a few short years away from becoming President of the Goddamn Universe. Less than 10 is simply unacceptable and should not be tolerated.

Welcome to the shallow world of pageantry as your baby endures his first real-world test for success and riches. It's a cruel world, so why not start the social ranking early, right? Right.

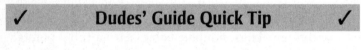

✓   Dudes' Guide Quick Tip   ✓

Don't confuse the Apgar test for newborns with the Ap-YARRR! test for pirate proficiency.

Delivery Notice

The classic waiting-room birth announcement can be simultaneously exhilarating and nerve-wracking, to say the least. Unless you're one of those caricature artists that you see on the boardwalk who can draw a hilariously big-headed charcoal portrait of mom and baby in an exaggerated, comical situation (e.g., mom holding baby while surfing), we highly recommend a digital camera in this situation. You can easily show pictures of the newborn to the anxiously curious mob of family and friends awaiting your appearance.

Be aware going in that you'll probably be bombarded with a whole bunch of questions you can't answer and will end up angering the crowd instead of enlightening them. In fact, when Scott's daughter was born, his experience with telling the group that had congregated in the waiting room was eerily similar to a White House press briefing you might catch on C-SPAN. We hope the following transcription of the video of Scott's actual briefing proves useful to your experience:

Scott: [enters the waiting room] Good morning, ladies and gentlemen. I realize it's been a long night for all of us. I will be making a brief statement and will have time to answer a few questions afterward. At approximately 7:47 this morning, Grace Katherine Finch was born via vaginal delivery. Shortly thereafter, it was determined that she weighed 8 pounds, 15 ounces and was 20.1 inches in length. The infant in question is healthy, pink, bald, and adorable, as far as the medical team was able to determine with the information that was available to them. Her mother wishes to express her gratitude for your support throughout this process, and I would personally like to echo those sentiments.

At this time, I will take a few brief questions. Umm, yes, Mom?

Scott's mom: How long did she have to push?

Scott: The baby had descended into the birth canal at approximately 5:20 a.m., which puts the actual pushing time at just under two and a half hours.

Scott's sister-in-law: Does the baby look like me?

Scott: As I stated in my opening remarks, it has been determined that the baby does exhibit traits that are consistent with what may be considered "cute," but at this time, we're not able to go into any details regarding, for example, whose nose the baby has. However, you can rest assured the baby does indeed have a nose, at least until Grandpa manages to steal it. [Smattering of laughter]

Scott's brother: Is the baby messed up at all?

Scott: I believe you're referring to any obvious birth defects, of which there were none that were immediately visible, aside from a misshapen head due to the time spent in the birth canal.

Scott's grandfather: Are his balls huge?

Scott: The baby is a girl, Grandpa.

Scott's dad: This is a two-part question: 1. What color is the baby's hair? and 2. What, if any, traits may be similar to the mother or father?

Scott: Again, these are both questions that I either can't address at this time or have already addressed. I won't be able to go into any further details.

Scott's dad: Just answer the question!

Scott: [flustered] I-I will in due time.

Scott's dad: You're clearly dodging the—

Scott: I have time for one more question. Yes, Aunt Patty.

Aunt Patty: How bad did her vagina tear?

Scott: Okay, that's all the time we have for questions now. I'll be sure to pass on additional information as it becomes available to us. Thanks again for your patience.

[Scott hurriedly leaves the room as the crowd continues to shout questions]: "When can we see her?"; "Does she look like me?"; "How long are her arms?"; etc.

Parental Notification Too

Beside the members of the press corps in the waiting room, there are many more (normal) friends and family members going about their day-to-day business who want to know the birth details. Word has probably gotten out that you checked into the hospital a day or so ago and now, depending on the laws of the state you live in, you may be criminally and civilly liable if you don't pass along the pertinent baby information as soon as reasonably possible.

Just as sensitive as the information and the timetable of the spreading of said information is, so is the order in which the information is spread. Fortunately, you've had practice here, or at least managed to fuck up the Wedding Table Approach once already. If so, it's time for redemption. If you've thought ahead (and you haven't), grab your chart of wedding table assignments from your wedding reception that you (should have learned to) keep with you at all times. This, once again, is the exact order in which you need to inform those wedding guests about the arrival of the new baby. The questions you will need to answer:

- "What is the baby's name?" If you get this wrong, score yourself a big 0 on your first standardized fatherhood test.
- "What is the baby's gender?" 95 percent of the time, this question will be answered by the name question. (Note: "Gender" means boy or girl.)
- "How much did the baby weigh?" You'll need to be accurate to the ounce. It's not like your wife's fat friend is going to challenge you about the proper weight, but in the future, if they're having a conversation about your 7-pound, 8-ounce baby and chubsy says, "But Bill told me it was 7 pounds, *9 ounces!*" you'll be in for a completely unavoidable, completely useless argument. Note: Additional questions will need to be addressed if the baby weighs less than 6 pounds ("Was your wife

shooting heroin during the pregnancy?") or more than
8.5 pounds ("Did your wife survive the delivery?").

- ■ "How long was he/she?" This is like weight in that
  you have to be accurate. Otherwise, even your standard midget clocks in at 19 or so inches at birth.

- ■ "How long was she in labor/did she have to push?" Only
  females are interested in this. You will be required to listen to the especially annoying ones tell you right then and
  there that they were in labor/pushed for much longer.

- ■ "How is the mother doing?" "She's fine but very tired"
  is the standard answer. No need for elaboration about
  tearing, cutting, bleeding, etc. The time for healing
  (for you) has begun.

- ■ "How's the baby?" Bill actually used the expression
  "She seems cool" when asked this question. Bill thought
  it perfectly summed up what the baby was like—her de-
  meanor, cuteness factor, etc. Bill is still getting yelled
  at for saying that. The Dudes suggest you find something better to say.

Repeat ten to ninety-seven times for other phone calls.

A practical way to avoid having to talk to all your wife's
annoying friends is to designate a friend to notify everybody, as you will be too busy worrying about being the
worst dad ever (and you're probably right). This should be
a trusted friend of your wife, not you. Your stupid friends
will hardly be able to remember the baby's first name and
are only vaguely aware of what an "ounce" is in non-steak-
related situations. A trusted friend of your wife can pass
along phone calls or e-mails to three friends who in turn
can forward the message to three more friends and on and

on until Bill Gates sends you $1,000, and the Taco Bell dog jumps across your computer screen, offering you a free trip to Disneyland if you press F8 for six seconds.

On the Mark

Can you imagine anything more adorable than your baby being born with something called a "stork bite" or an "angel kiss?" Who doesn't love being kissed by an angel or bitten by a stork?

Well, you should know that our friend Mike was once involved in a horrific incident involving a fish sandwich and a stork, and let's just say Mike won't be visiting the Everglades anytime soon without a handgun. It just goes to show, you shouldn't be fooled by doctor's placating you with cutesy terms in reference to skin abnormalities. Sure, kissing an angel sounds nice, but next thing you know, it's escalated to banging the angel once a week at the Howard Johnson, and now she's threatening to tell everybody if you don't leave your wife for her. We're just saying, is all.

Birthmarks are almost entirely harmless, medically speaking. Stork bites/angel kisses usually fade within a year, while others, like the adorably nicknamed strawberry, blue bum, café au lait, or port-wine stain are gifts for life. Facial birthmarks can be cause for psychological concern, but let's put it in perspective here. It's only a psychological concern for you. Your baby doesn't give a crap if he's got a mark on his face, and by the time he's old enough for other asshole kids to tease him about it, surgical intervention will help calm *your* nerves.

Antiskin and Foreskin

As you know, the wiener is a mysterious and troublesome beast. Having a boy only compounds the problem. With a boy, you'll be forced to decide whether or not to have his foreskin surgically hacked off by the doctor.

There are a myriad of arguments about why it's cruel and unnecessary. "They" say it causes trauma and stress for both the baby and the parents. "They" say it decreases sexual sensitivity later in life. "They" say it changes sleep and activity patterns. "They" say a bunch of other ridiculous crap about why circumcision should be avoided at birth and left up to the individual to decide later.

Well, The Dudes think that "they" can go suck it. "They" are usually the same people who are loath to give pain medication to women during childbirth and will do anything it takes to deliver vaginally, or "naturally." While The Dudes are also proponents of vaginal birth, it's for purely aesthetic reasons. Yes, we know, we're horrible, horrible people.

With all the circumcision controversy swirling around, we've decided to take a stand. The Dudes' official position regarding the foreskin is as firm as our members, and it is as follows:

The foreskin sucks.

We can't remember a single day in our lives when we looked down and said, "Man, I really miss my foreskin, and I'll never forgive my parents for fucking up my entire life." We can't remember ever wishing we had an extra 12 square inches of loose skin hanging off the tip of our units.

There are no rock ballads that we know of written about foreskin loss and the heartbreak that follows. The last thing we want to do is push our skin sock out of the way in order to actually accomplish tasks.

Foreskin lovers would tell us that it's not about superficial issues or even convenience. It's really about choice. Some men who miss their foreskins actually join support groups to talk about their issues with being "robbed" of said foreskins.

The Dudes unabashedly mock and belittle these men. "How can you feel comfortable making this painful, medically unnecessary choice for your boy?" they ask. Well, in accordance with our official position about the foreskin completely sucking, we're well prepared to mock and belittle our own boys if they even think of joining a foreskin-loss support group.

Helpful Advice

Now, more than ever, you might be freaking out about how you're going to be able to handle all the stress of your job along with the stress of a new baby and a recovering wife. Sorry, dude.

Check Her Out

There was a time when if your wife wasn't bleeding profusely from her vagina, the hospital would send the lot of you home to make way for more little dollar signs—er, we mean women in labor. Now, laws often dictate how long you'll be staying at the hospital, which is typically a full calendar day *after* the day the baby is delivered, checking out the morning after that. Bill's wife delivered at 12:20 a.m. on a Wednesday, providing for an all-expenses-paid, two-day stay at the Hotel Presbyterian, complete with three free 2-star meals a day, adjustable bed, and complimentary babysitting services.

The recovery period involves constant visits from nurses, obstetricians, pediatricians, lactation consultants, baby photographers, baby photo studio representatives, timeshare salespeople, and housekeepers. It will also involve you running errands for your wife between reruns of *Everybody Loves Raymond* on TV in the hospital room.

This actually helps prepare you for years of running errands for your wife between reruns of *Everybody Loves Raymond* on TV at home. This postdelivery period may be the most peaceful time in what is an entirely new experience for you called parenthood. The Dudes advise you to take every advantage available to you, especially the nursery. At home, you won't have nurses with years of experience awake twenty-four hours a day to take care of your screaming child. That is, if you don't count Nurse Wife, who will be awake for weeks at a time. What a trouper.

The hospital will probably give you some parting gifts, including huge, absorbent crotch pads, diapers, a baby blanket, and whatever else you manage to "accidentally" pack in your suitcase.

Many hospitals will have a nurse wheel your wife and new baby out of the hospital. This may seem like a kind "It's been nice having you" gesture, but rest assured, the hospital maintains a strict "don't let the door hit you on the way out" attitude. The nurse is accompanying your family to the car to make sure you strap your newborn into an approved infant car seat. "Awww," you think, "that's sweet that they're concerned about the baby's safety." More accurately, it's more of an, "Awww, they're making sure the baby's strapped in so the hospital doesn't get sued if we get in an accident."

With the hospital in your rearview mirror, you'll inevitably get that empty feeling that you're now on your own. We would like to take this opportunity to point out that not only is the hospital done helping you, but so are we. The advice gravy train has reached the mashed potato station, and it's time to unload. It's not because we don't know or care, it's just that we've already helped you so damn much, and this is all the advice you're going to get for $12. Much like the hospital, though, we're always gonna be there for you if you need us, as long as the cash keeps coming.

📖 **Myth vs. Fact** 📖

Myth: Every birth is a miracle.
Fact: Miracles, by definition, do not involve vaginal tearing.

Myth: Your coworkers can be a great resource for your pregnancy-related questions.
Fact: Your foreign coworkers can be a great source of comedy.

Myth: Your doctor will help you through labor, delivery, and recovery.
Fact: Your doctor will walk into the delivery room in time to catch the baby and collect his fee.

A.D.

After Delivery

The weeks following the baby's delivery are wrought with discoveries of just how inept you are at being a father, which will conveniently help you forget how inept you were at being a father-to-be. But don't move on too quickly. The Dudes would like to take a moment to reflect on the last nine-plus months of terror and how you may not have done so badly after all. Remember that whole means-to-an-end thing we mentioned earlier? This is the end result. You're at home with a baby, and there's a good chance the baby hasn't discovered that you're an asshole yet. So you best get in some quality time before he or she learns your not-so-dark secret.

Your wife has already forgotten about the pain of delivery, but it's probably a result of her being preoccupied with the pain of recovery. And though your crotch isn't bleeding (it shouldn't be), you should take some time to recover as well. You've been to hell and back.

You could look back on the weeks of robo-fucking that led to her missing period and pregnancy test, followed by weeks of puking, nausea, and boob pain as a precursor to dizziness and food cravings; before her jeans became too tight and she cried all the time, farting her way to her belly expansion and butt growth, making way for the ultrasound and fight over names, predating the baby shower and maternity class; along with her newfound stretch marks, enlarged boobs, and leaky genitals; making for awkward, uncomfortable sex that culminated in uncomfortable sleep; useless labor-induction techniques; false labor; mucus plug; water breaking on your couch; painful contractions; perilous drive to the hospital; pain chart; dilation; epidural; and actual delivery.

But try not to dwell on it too much—that stuff wasn't all her fault. Instead, The Dudes suggest you take some time to admire your heroism over the last several months. You didn't let her crying bring you down, her nausea make you weary, her discharge make you cringe. Well, at least you triumphed over most of those things.

But why dwell on the misery of the past when you can contemplate the suffering of the future?

- When will his crusty, black belly button extension fall off?
- When will she get her first ear infection?
- When will he swallow his first quarter?
- When will she learn how to curse?
- When will he experience the awkwardness of puberty?
- When will she fall in love with some asshole?

Instead, The Dudes recommend that you grab a glass of vodka, one of your wife's prescription painkillers, and live right now,[1] because right now is pretty good: your elated, triumphant wife; your beautiful, sleeping baby; your kick-ass chair; and a Vico-tini temporarily suppressing utter panic.

Hey, it's not like we ever said this was going to be easy.

---

1. The Dudes' legal team has advised against us recommending mixing vodka and painkillers.

Glossary

Apgar: Your baby's first permanent record of imperfection

The Big Scar: Imperfection following Caesarian section (C-section) delivery

The Big Snip: Episiotomy

bloody show: Heavy spotting coinciding with labor. The grossest term ever

Brain Window: Small, skull-free area on your baby's head

Braxton Hicks contractions: Uterine weight lifting

breaking the popsicle: Massage technique performed just like it sounds

cervix: *see* wombhole

changing table: Specially designed table for changing your baby's diaper. Waaaay better than a regular table, floor, or other flat surface

Chinese fertility chart: Gender test based on an ancient Asian chart. Approximately 50 percent accurate

couples shower: A baby shower that men are invited to. They are also invited to punch your dick

DICs: Dudes in Cubes. Scott's advice-prone coworkers at Condor Global Logistics Mega Corp

dilation and effacement: 1. Opening and thinning of the cervix, respectively; early labor indicators of a baby's delivery progress 2. Popular lesbian folk duo

divine abortion: Miscarriage

Doctor-Nurse Dynamic: Medical equivalent of Marx's bourgeoisie-proletariat dynamic

Drano test: Gender test utilizing Drano drain unclogger. Approximately 50 percent accurate

The Dudes: Bill Lloyd, Scott Finch, and any other kick-ass males who are looking out for you

foreskin: Most useless flap of wiener skin ever to inspire a social movement

Great Big Fat Person: Great big unwanted advice-giver

The Great Realization: Your father-in-law's all-too-real discovery that you're banging his daughter

Groundhog Day effect: A negative pregnancy test resulting in three to four weeks of frustration for your wife

hemorrhoids: Itchy, enlarged anal butt veins

High School Factor: The probability of one's name being used as an insult

Hyatt Humping: Carefree intercourse in a hotel room

lanugo: Baby fur. Can fetch upwards of $500 an ounce

linea nigra: Literally "black line." Possibly permanent, unattractive vertical abdominal line resulting from pregnancy

lotus birth: Birth process in which the umbilical cord and placenta are not severed after birth but are allowed to naturally decay away. Popular in countries with few scissors/knives

Lucky Hotness: The unlikely increase in attractiveness after pregnancy

meconium: Fetus poo

The Metamorphosis: The unlikely event of a pregnant woman becoming a MILF

MILF (Mom I'd Like to Fuck): A female—with children—with whom one would enjoy vigorous intercourse

Montgomery Glands: Leaky nipple bumps usually found on inexpensive strippers

mystery bag: A shared bag of maternity clothes that friends and family trade/add to during their respective pregnancies

National Geographic specials: 1. Popular series of educational television programs in the 1980s. 2. Saggy boobs

Ninja's Revenge: Unspeakable sexual position

nursery: A term used to describe your baby's room to make it sound like it's more than just a room for the baby to sleep in

pencil test: Gender test in which a pencil tied to a string is suspended over a pregnant woman's stomach. Approximately 50 percent accurate

perineum: Taint

Pitocin: Magic labor-inducing potion rumored to be made from hemlock and the tears of the innocent

placenta: Uterine meat pocket

pork: To have intercourse with

port-wine stain: Gorby-style birthmark

Post-Pregnancy Hotness Recovery: The ability of a pregnant woman to regain her prepregnancy attractiveness

Pregnancy Watch: Anticipatory period of heightened awareness by a woman's friends and family brought on by a miscarriage

pushing: The active stage of crapping out a kid

reproba verum: A comforting half-truth. From the Latin for "false truth"

robo-fucking: Frequent, mechanical intercourse for the purpose of conceiving a child

rotating metal disk test: Made-up gender test utilizing a flipped coin. Approximately 50 percent accurate

Scrotum Falls: Testicles

sex in an envelope: Your baby's gender written secretly on a piece of paper for you and your wife to discover together after an ultrasound

sleepfarts: Nighttime episodes of flatulence during pregnancy

SOS (Sexual Oasis of Sex): A brief period of intense intercourse during the fourth month of pregnancy

spank bank: The area of the brain that stores pornographic images for masturbatory purposes

Steak-a-saurus: Oversized novelty sirloin that can't be eaten by the average man

stretch marks: Purplish lines on the abdomen, buttocks, and legs. Your child's certificate of authenticity

trying: Prepregnancy period of robo-fucking

vaginal sneeze: The ejection of the mucus plug. A gross sign of labor

vernix: Technical term for a newborn's goo coating

Vico-tini: Hydrocodone/vodka cocktail

water birth: A birth in a vat of uterine goo and chunks

Wedding Table Approach: Announcing pregnancy in the order of proximity of wedding guests to the head table at your wedding

"We're pregnant": Required declaration of pregnancy, especially when your spouse is nearby

wombhole: *see* cervix

your mom: The biggest whore we know

Index